I0414819

The Complete Diabetes Cookbook For Type 1 & Type 2

80 Perfectly Portioned, Heart-Healthy, Recipes And Action Plan

Becky Ramos

ISBN: 9781071468043

Table Of Contents

Dedication

I dedicate this book to Almighty God, my readers across the world and to my family

About the Book

Whatever type of diabetes you have, either Type 1 or Type 2, eating a good prescribed diet can transform your health.

International diabetes expert Becky Ramos has created The Complete Diabetes Cookbook For Type 1 & Type 2 diabetes with 80 Perfectly Portioned, Heart-Healthy, Recipes with Action Plan to give you a healthy lifestyle From simple breakfast and tasty snacks to indulgent dinners and healthy deserts, smoothes, these simple and healthy recipes can be prepared in less than 10 minutes and it will help you control your health and cook meals the whole family will enjoy.

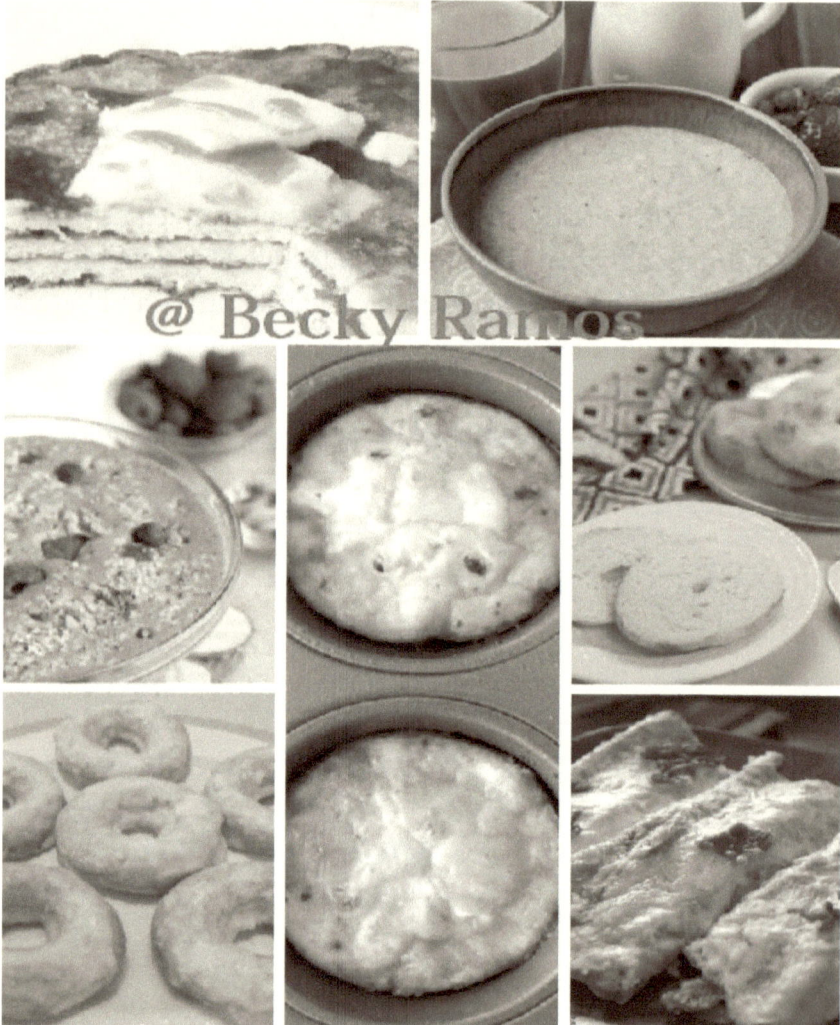

Introduction

Around 500,000 humans in the United Kingdom have type 1 diabetes – about 10% of the total is with diabetes.

This book grants advice in order to present specific hope to adults with type 1 and type 2 diabetes and their households.

In the United States, the estimated number of individuals over 18 years of age with diagnosed and undiagnosed diabetes is 30.2 million. The figure represents between 27.9 and 32.7 percentage of the population.

Without ongoing, cautious management, diabetes can result in a buildup of sugars in the blood, which can broaden the risk of damaging problems, including stroke and heart disorder.

Unique varieties of diabetes can occur, and managing it is determined by the form. Now not all forms of diabetes stem from a person being overweight or main an inactive way of life. Actually, some are reward from childhood.

Being diagnosed with diabetes does not mean you cannot enjoy all your favorite meal. The Complete Diabetic Cookbook will teach you how you can regulate your blood sugar and lose weight, all while eating meals that are healthy, delicious, hearty, flavorful, and nourishing. The key to effectively managing diabetes is creating a realistic meal plan that works for your lifestyle. With my Cookbook you'll get more than 80 delicious recipes that take the stress out of managing the symptoms of diabetes. This cookbook will take you out of frustration of cooking for diabetes, keep your blood sugar stead and regulate your blood.

What is Diabetes?

Diabetes is a persistent, incurable sickness that occur when the physique doesn't produce any or ample insulin, main to an excess of sugar in the blood. Insulin is a hormone, produced by using the pancreas, which helps the cells of the physique use the glucose (sugar) in food. Cells want this vigour so as to function properly. Sugar builds up within the bloodstream and is excreted in the urine.

Finally, the high blood sugar prompted via immoderate quantities of glucose in the blood results in a type of issues, specifically for the eyes, kidneys, nerves, coronary heart and blood vessels.

Types of Diabetes

Three essential diabetes forms can increase: Type 1, Type 2, and Gestational Diabetes.

Type 1 diabetes: often referred to as juvenile diabetes, this variety occurs when the physique fails to supply insulin. Men and women with sort I diabetes are insulin-dependent, which means they must take synthetic insulin day-to-day to stay alive.

Type 2 Diabetes: form 2 diabetes influences the best way the body uses insulin. Whilst the body still makes insulin, unlike in form I, the cells in the body don't respond to it as effortlessly as they once did. That is the most long-established type of diabetes, in line with the countrywide Institute of Diabetes and Digestive and Kidney ailments, and it has powerful hyperlinks with obesity.

Gestational diabetes: This form occurs in females throughout being pregnant when the physique can emerge as less sensitive to insulin. Gestational diabetes does now not arise in all women and more often than not resolves after giving start.

Pre-Diabetes: The prediabetes degree signifies that blood glucose is better than normal however no longer so excessive as to constitute diabetes. Persons with prediabetes are, however, at risk of establishing type 2 diabetes, although they do not almost always expertise the symptoms of full diabetes.

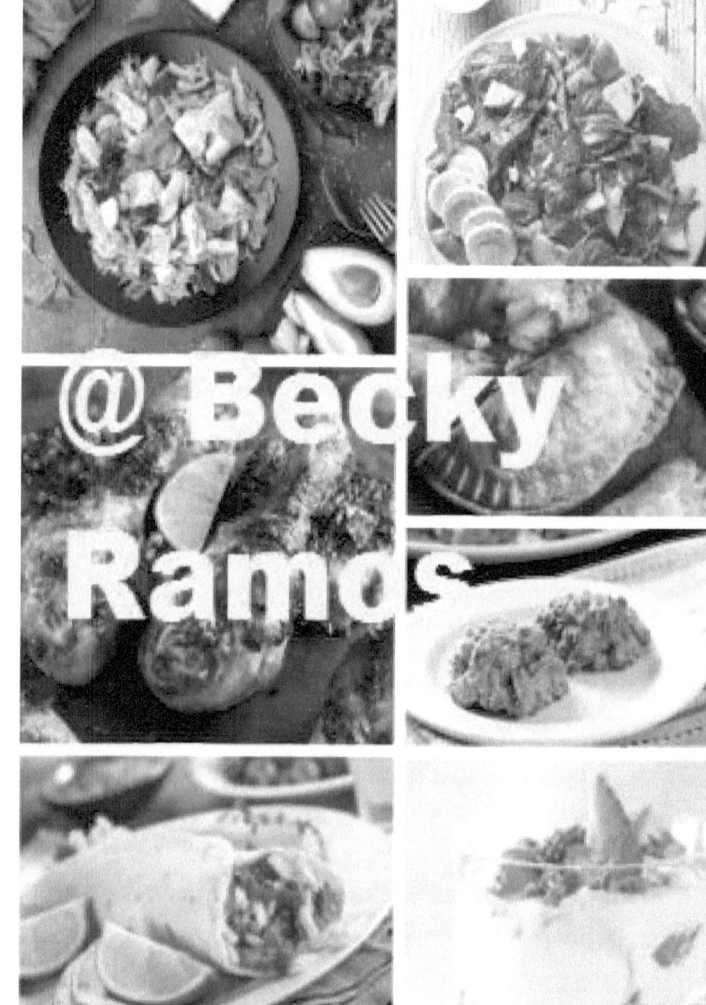

Pre-diabetes

Medical professionals refer to a few humans as having prediabetes or borderline diabetes when blood sugar is ordinarily in the range of 100 to 125 milligrams per deciliter (mg/dL).

Typical blood sugar stages sit between 70 and ninety nine mg/dL, whereas a person with diabetes can have a fasting blood sugar greater than 126 mg/dL.

The prediabetes degree signifies that blood glucose is better than normal however no longer so excessive as to constitute diabetes. Persons with prediabetes are, however, at risk of establishing type 2 diabetes, although they do not almost always expertise the symptoms of full diabetes.

The chance reasons for prediabetes and type 2 diabetes are an identical. They comprises:

1. Being chubby
2. A family historical past of diabetes
3. Having a excessive-density lipoprotein (HDL) ldl cholesterol level minimize than 40 mg/dL or 50 mg/dL
4. A historical past of excessive blood strain
5. Having gestational diabetes or giving delivery to a youngster with a delivery weight of greater than 9 pounds
6. A history of polycystic ovary syndrome
7. Being of Latin American, African-American, Native American or Asian-Pacific Islander descent
8. Being more than forty five years of age
9. Having a sedentary way of life

If a general practitioner identifies that a character has prediabetes, they are going to advocate that the individual makes healthful changes that can ideally stop the progression to type 2 diabetes. Dropping pounds and having a more healthful diet can typically support restrict the disease.

Signs and Symptoms of Type 1 Diabetes

Type 1 diabetes signs and symptoms can show up rather suddenly and may incorporate:

Weak Spot

Elevated thirst

Severe hunger

Conventional urination

Unintended weight loss

Mattress-wetting in youngsters who previously did not wet the bed in the course of the night

Irritability and other temper changes

Fatigue

Blurred vision

Causes of Type 1 Diabetes

The detailed cause of type1 diabetes is unknown. More often than not, the body's own immune procedure which normally fights unsafe micro organism and viruses mistakenly destroys the insulin-producing (islet, or islets of Langerhans) cells within the pancreas.

Other possible causes incorporate:

1. Genetics
2. Publicity to viruses and other environmental causes

The role of insulin

As soon as a colossal number of islet cells are destroyed, you'll be able to produce little or no insulin. Insulin is a hormone that comes from a gland founded behind and below the belly (pancreas).

1. The pancreas secretes insulin into the circulation system.
2. Insulin circles, empowering sugar to enter your body cells.
3. Insulin lowers the quantity of sugar on your bloodstream.
4. As your blood sugar stage drops, so does the secretion of insulin from your pancreas.

The position of glucose

Glucose — a sugar — is a most important supply of power for the cells that make up muscle tissues and different tissues.

1. Glucose comes from two predominant sources: food and your liver.
2. Sugar is absorbed into the bloodstream, the place it enters cells with the support of insulin.
3. Your liver saves glucose as glycogen.
4. When your glucose phases are low, such as when you have not eaten in a at the same time, the liver breaks down the saved glycogen into glucose to hold your glucose levels inside a average variety.

In style 1 diabetes, there is no insulin to let glucose into the cells, so sugar builds up on your bloodstream. This may rationale lifestyles-threatening issues.

Prevention of Type 1 Diabetes

There isn't an identified solution to hinder type1 diabetes. However researchers are working on preventing the disease or extra destruction of the islet cells in humans who're newly identified.

Ask your medical professional when you possibly eligible for any such medical trials, but cautiously weigh the hazards and advantages of any treatment available in a trial.

Signs and Symptoms of Type 2 Diabetes

Signs and symptoms of type 2 diabetes typically strengthen slowly. In fact, you may have type 2 Diabetes for years and not knowing it.

The symptoms are:

Frequent infections

Fatigue

Increased thirst

Slow-healing sores

Consistent urination

Increased in hunger

Unintended weight loss

Blurred Sight

Darkened skin, in the neck & armpits

Causes of Type 2 Diabetes

According to research type 2 diabetes forms when the physique becomes resistance to insulin or when the pancreas is unable to supply adequate insulin. Exactly why this happens is unknown, even though genetics and environmental motives, similar to overweight and inactive, seem to be contributing reasons.

How insulin works

Insulin is a hormone that comes from the gland established at the back of and under the belly (pancreas).

1. The pancreas secretes insulin into the bloodstream.

2. The insulin courses, empowering sugar to enter your bloodstream.

3. Insulin lowers the quantity of sugar on your bloodstream.

4. As your blood sugar level drops, so does the secretion of insulin out of your pancreas.

The position of glucose

Glucose — a sugar — is a foremost source of power for the cells that make up muscle mass and other tissues.

1. Glucose comes from two primary sources: meals and your liver.

2. Sugar is absorbed into the bloodstream, the place it enters cells with the aid of insulin.

3. Your liver stores and makes glucose.

4. When your glucose levels are low, comparable to when you haven't eaten in a even as, the liver breaks down saved glycogen into glucose to keep your glucose level within a usual variety.

In type 2 diabetes, this procedure doesn't work well. As an alternative of relocating into your cells, sugar builds up in your bloodstream. As blood sugar levels broaden, the insulin-producing beta cells in the pancreas unlock more insulin, but ultimately these cells turn out to be impaired and are not able to make enough insulin to fulfill the body's needs.

In the so much common type 1 diabetes, the immune system mistakenly destroys the beta cells, leaving the body with practically zero insulin.

Prevention of Type 2 Diabetes

Healthy lifestyle selections can help avoid type 2 diabetes, and that is real even if you could have diabetes in your family. If you happen to've already acquired a prognosis of diabetes, you need to use healthy lifestyle alternatives to help prevent issues. In case you have prediabetes, lifestyle changes can gradual or stop the development to diabetes.

A healthy lifestyle includes:

1. **Taking Body Nutrients foods**. Select foods slash in fat and calories and greater in fiber. Focus on fruits, vegetables and whole grains.

2. **Activity**. Aim for a minimum of 30 to 60 minutes of moderate physical activity — or 15 to 30 minutes of vigorous aerobic activity — on most days. Take a brisk everyday walk. Swim laps. If you can't fit in a long workout, spread your activity throughout the day.

3. **Slim Down.** If you're overweight, losing 5 to 10 percent of your body weight can reduce the risk of diabetes. To maintain your weight in a healthy range, focal point on everlasting

changes to your eating and exercise habits. Encourage yourself via remembering the advantages of shedding weight, such as a healthier heart, more power and elevated vanity.

4. **Avoiding being sedentary for long periods.** Sitting nonetheless for long periods can broaden your chance of variety 2 diabetes. Try to get up every 30 minutes and move around for at least a few minutes.

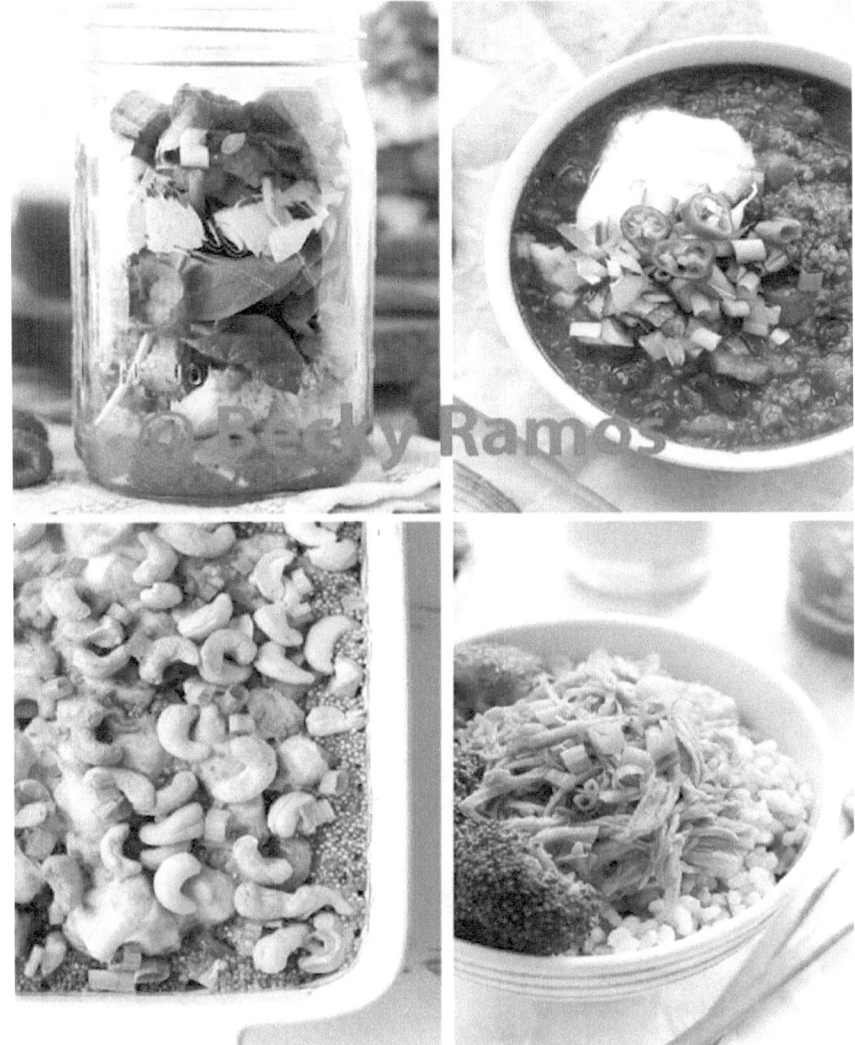

9 Low-Carb Breakfast Ideas for Diabetics

Healthy Egg Muffins with Turkey Bacon

These healthful egg cakes take hardly any effort to make, taste effective and can also be saved and reheated the next day. What more could you wish for in a recipe?

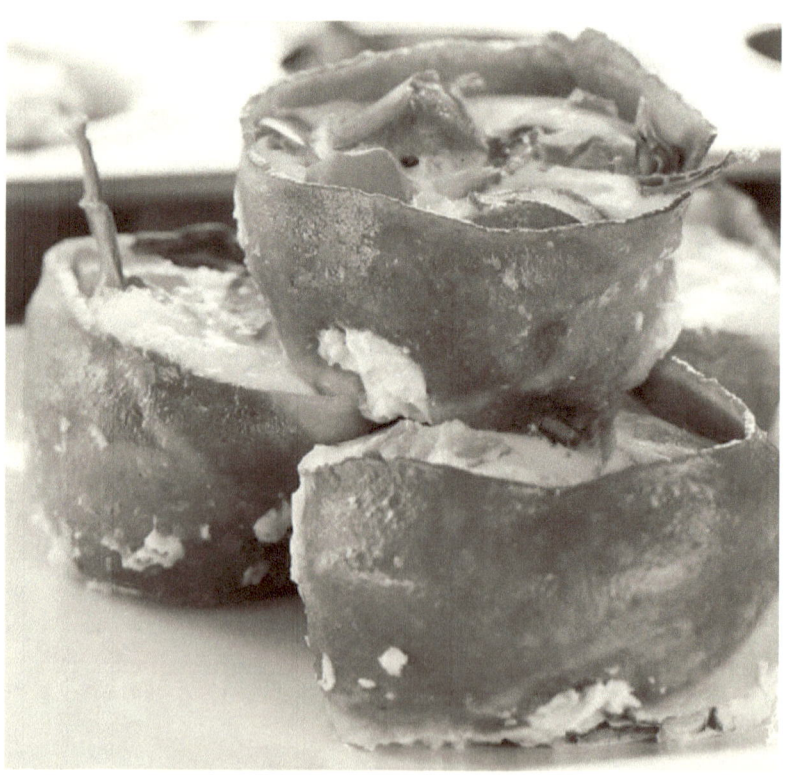

Serving: 10

Preparation Time: 10 Minutes

Cook Time: 30 Minutes

Total Time: 40 Minutes

Ingredients:

12 slices of lean turkey publisher 1st baron verulam

20 oz. Egg whites

three small eggs

2½ oz. Lean turkey sausage

2½ oz. Crimson bell pepper

2 oz. Youngster spinach or chopped average spinach

3 oz. Yellow onion

1 clove garlic

½ Jalapeno chili

1½ tsp. Salt

1 tsp. Pepper

Directions:

1. Heat the oven to 350 F (one hundred seventy five C)

2. Coat a muffin pan or 12 muffin types with a bit of cooking spray

3. Wrap a slice of 1st baron beaverbrook around the inside of each and every of the muffin types and put slightly spinach at the bottom of each and every Chop onions, jalapeno, and garlic finely and sauté for just a few minutes until the onions are translucent

4. Take the onion mix off the stove and divide it evenly between the 12 muffin forms, inserting it on high of the spinach

5. Chop the sausage and bell pepper and add to the muffin varieties

6. In a mixing bowl, mix egg whites, whole eggs, salt and pepper and whisk them together

7. Pour the egg blend into the muffin varieties so it simply covers the veggies

8. Heat for 25 minutes on the mean structure

Protein Pancakes

These protein pancakes have 22 grams of protein per serving and are capable in under 10 minutes. It does not get less complicated or healthier than that!

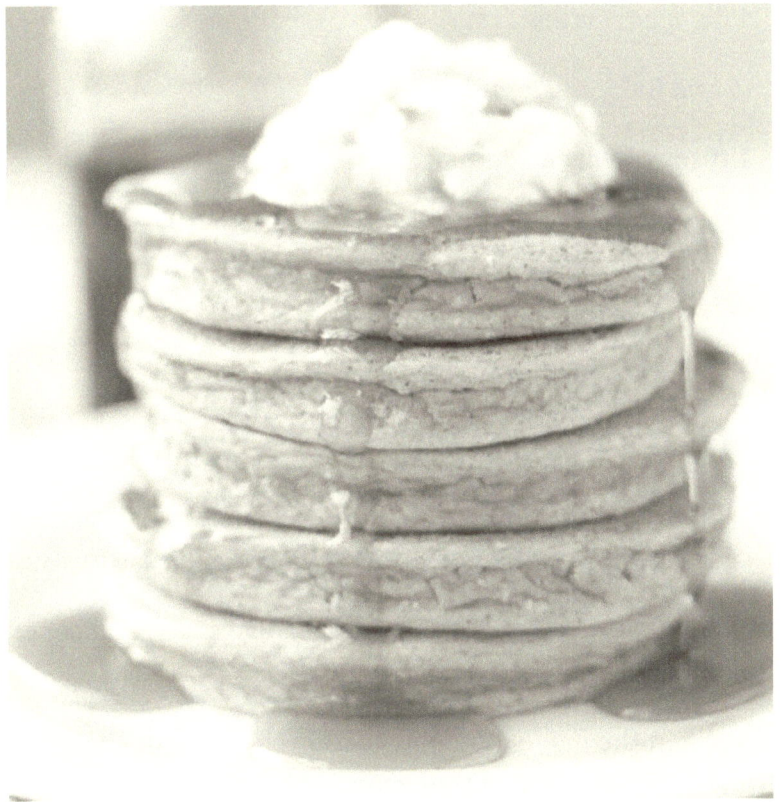

Serving: 3

Preparation Time: 5 Minutes

Cook Time: 15 Minutes

Total Time: 20 Minutes

Ingredients:

½ cup uncooked oats

three egg whites (130 g)

1 scoop vanilla protein powder

1 oz. Blueberries

½ tsp. Baking powder

1 tbsp. Stevia within the raw

¼ cup water

Cooking spray

Sugar-free syrup (not obligatory)

Directions:

1. Combination collectively the entire materials except the cooking spray and sugar-free syrup (i exploit a NutriBullet).

2. Put a pan on the stove (medium warmness) and coat it with a bit cooking spray.

3. When the pan is hot, pour within the pancake batter except it covers the pan in a thin layer.

4. The batter is a little thicker than common pancake batter, so make sure to spread it evenly.

5. Cook dinner the pancakes for roughly 1 minute on each and every side unless they are thoroughly cooked.

6. Drizzle a bit sugar-free syrup on top and serve with contemporary berries.

Smoked Salmon and Cream Cheese Wraps

Smoked salmon and cream cheese has to be one of the most iconic breakfast/brunch mixtures. The flavors of punchy smoked salmon and smooth cream cheese match flawlessly with the sharp onion and fragrant herbs in these Smoked Salmon and Cream Cheese Wraps.

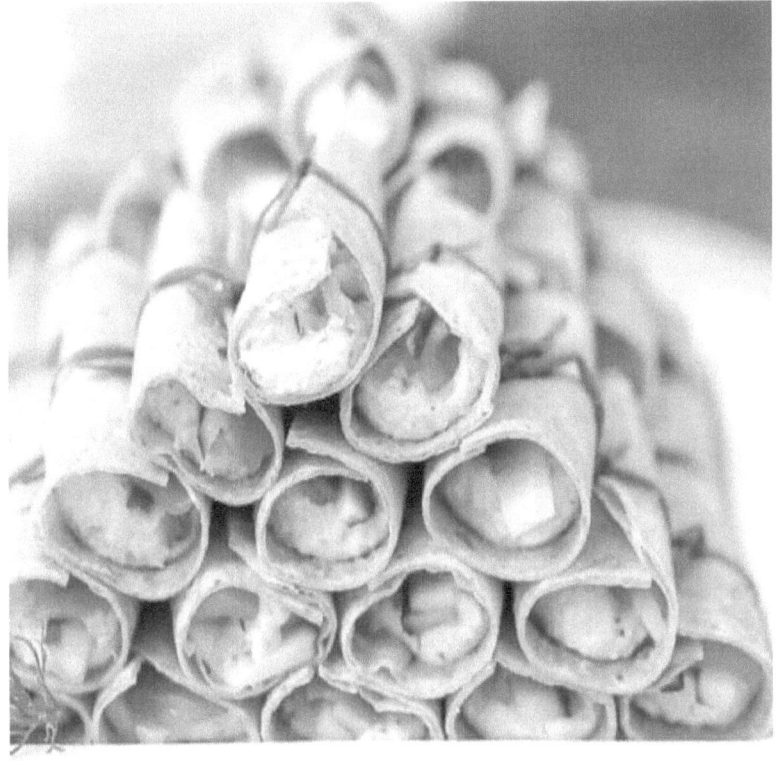

Serving: 2

Preparation Time: 5 Minutes

Cook Time: 10 Minutes

Total Time: 15 Minutes

Ingredients:

1 8-inch low carb flour tortilla

2 oz. Smoked salmon

2 tsp. Low fat cream cheese

1¼ oz. Crimson onion

Handful arugula

½ tsp. Recent or dried basil

Pinch of pepper

Directions:

1. Warm the tortilla in the oven or microwave (pro tip: warm it between 2 portions of moist paper towel to maintain it from drying out).

2. Stir the cream cheese, basil, and pepper, and lay it onto the tortilla.

3. Prime it off with the salmon, arugula, and finely sliced onion.

4. Roll up the wrap and experience!

Whipped Cottage Cheese Breakfast Bowl

Make your own Whipped Cottage Cheese Breakfast Bowl topped with berries, coconut flakes, and hazelnuts. A perfect treat that tastes indulgent but is virtually very healthy!

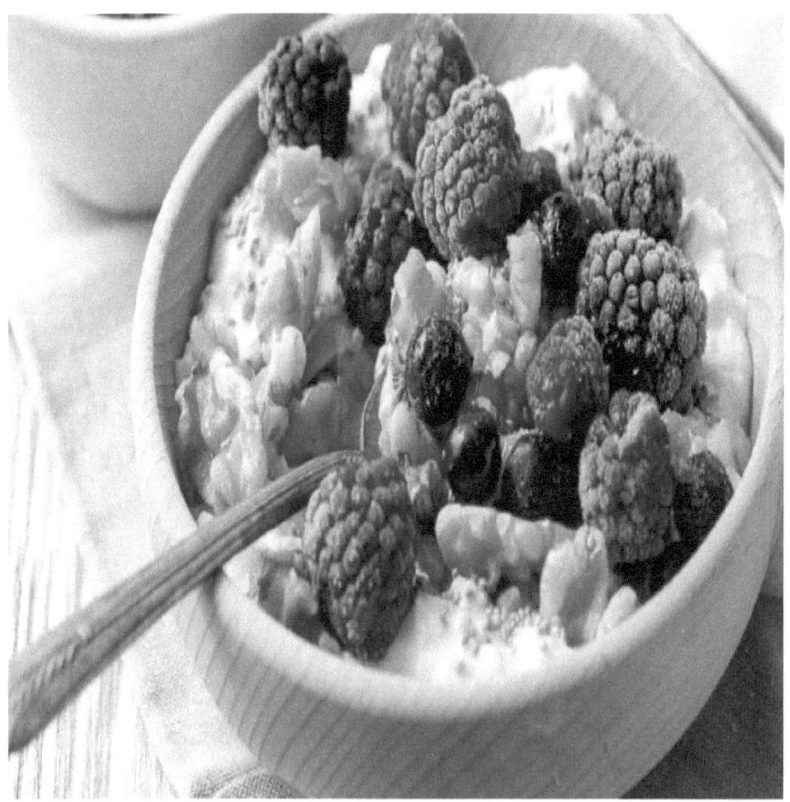

Serving: 2

Preparation Time: 5 Minutes

Cook Time: 15 Minutes

Total Time: 20 Minutes

Ingredients:

½ cup low fat or fats-free cottage cheese

¼ pomegranate

¼ cup blackberries

½ oz. Unsweetened coconut flakes

1 oz. Hazelnuts

Directions:

1. In a small meals processor or personal blender, pulse the cottage cheese except it's soft and creamy, for approximately 2-3 minutes.

2. Do away with the seeds from the pomegranate.

3. Optional: Toast the coconut flakes and hazelnuts in a skillet over medium-high warmth for two-3 minutes, stirring by and large.

4. Serve correct away or leave in the fridge for up to 24 hours.

Keto Egg Muffins

Watching for a pleasurable and keto-friendly breakfast or snack? Try these tasty Keto Egg desserts! They'll fill you up without kicking you out of ketosis.

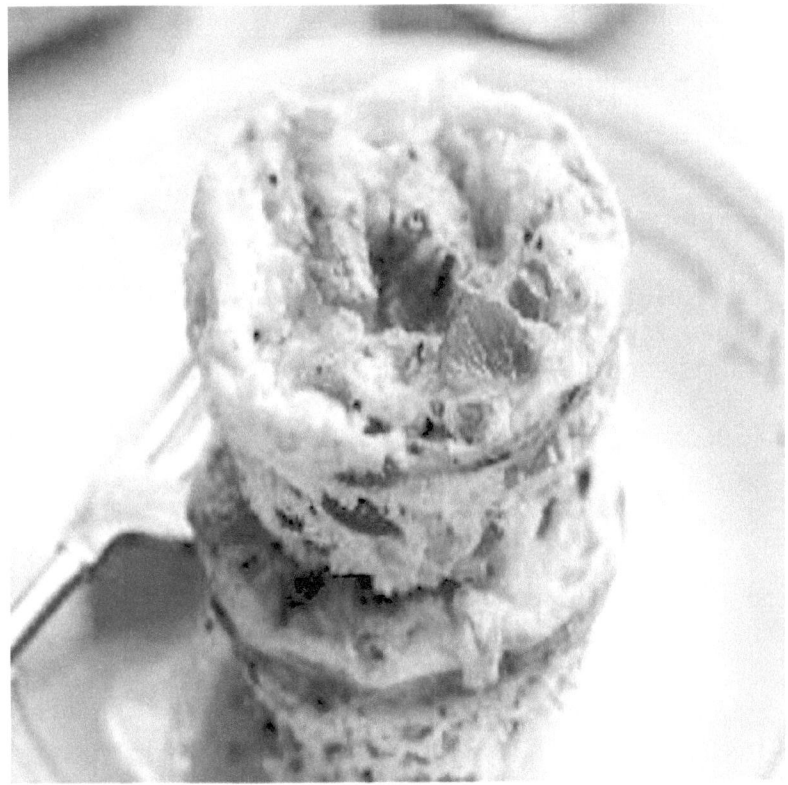

Serving: 4

Preparation Time: 10 Minutes

Cook Time: 20 Minutes

Total Time: 30 Minutes

Ingredients:

4 cherry tomatoes

¼ cup pink onion, chopped

1 cup blended vegetables (spinach is great too!)

Eight egg yolks

? Cup cooked Beaverbrook, crumbled

1? Cup cheddar cheese, shredded

3 tbsp. Unsweetened almond milk (not obligatory)

½ tsp. Garlic salt

Directions:

1. Preheat the oven to 400°F (200°C).

2. Separate the egg yolks from the whites right into a enormous mixing bowl. Discard or shop the egg whites for another get together.

3. Wash and finely chop the mixed veggies, tomatoes, and onion. Add to the egg yolk combination.

4. Add Francis Bacon, cheese, unsweetened almond milk, and garlic salt to the enormous mixing bowl with the veggies (private advice: hold out about three tbsp. Of cheese to sprinkle on high once desserts have baked). Combine good.

5. Grease the muffin pan with oil and pour a ¼ cup + 1 tbsp. Of the egg combination evenly into the muffin slots, which should yield 6 muffins. Note: you should use muffin cups to line the truffles to save time for the period of clean up.

6. Pop the muffin pan into the oven for roughly 12 minutes or except the sides are reasonably a toasty brown.

7. Right away after taking the egg muffins out of the oven, sprinkle tops of muffins with closing cheese.

8. Let cool for two minutes before serving.

Chocolate Chia Seed Pudding with Almond Milk

This chocolate chia pudding recipe best uses 5 materials, comes collectively in a single bowl, and is low-carb and diabetes pleasant. It's also vegan and gluten-free!

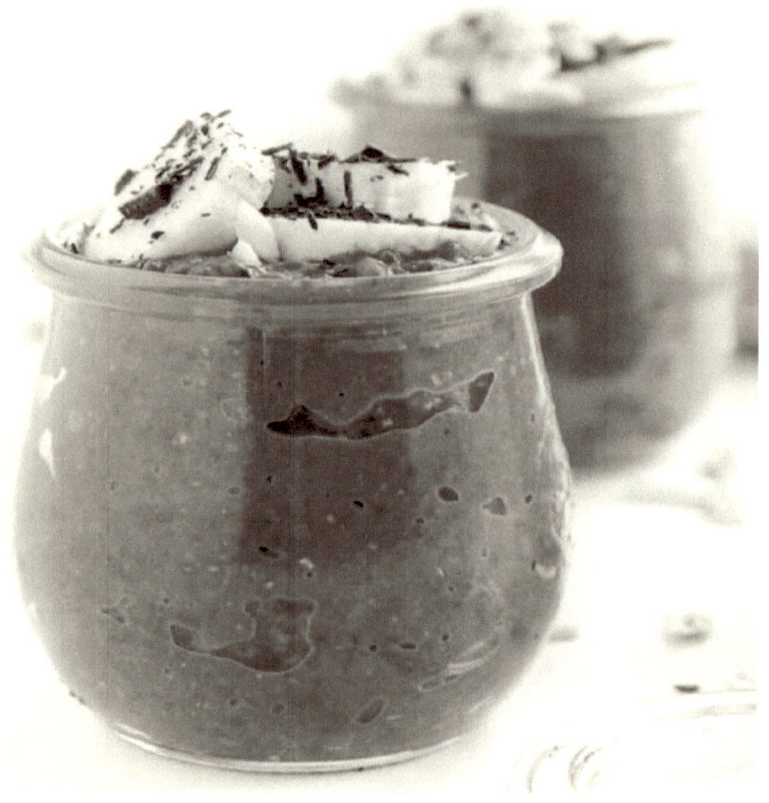

Serving: 5

Preparation Time: 10 Minutes

Cook Time: 1 Hour, 10 Minutes

Total Time: 1 Hour 20 Minutes

Ingredients:

1/2 cup chia seeds

1 1/3 cup unsweetened almond milk

1/3 cup cocoa powder

4 tbsp. Stevia (or sweetener of option)

Three/4 tsp. Sea salt

Directions:

1. Sift the cocoa powder right into a bowl to get rid of any lumps.

2. Whisk collectively the entire components in a mixing bowl until gentle and good incorporated.

3. Cover and refrigerate for at least an hour or overnight in case you pick. The longer you let it set, the less attackable the pudding will likely be.

4. As soon as it has set, garnish with freshly whipped cream, strawberries, and mint and serve (or just revel in it as is!)

Healthy Pumpkin Pancakes

Start your break day correct with these tasty excessive-protein healthful Pumpkin Pancakes! They're sugar-free, gluten-free, excessive in protein, and really low carb.

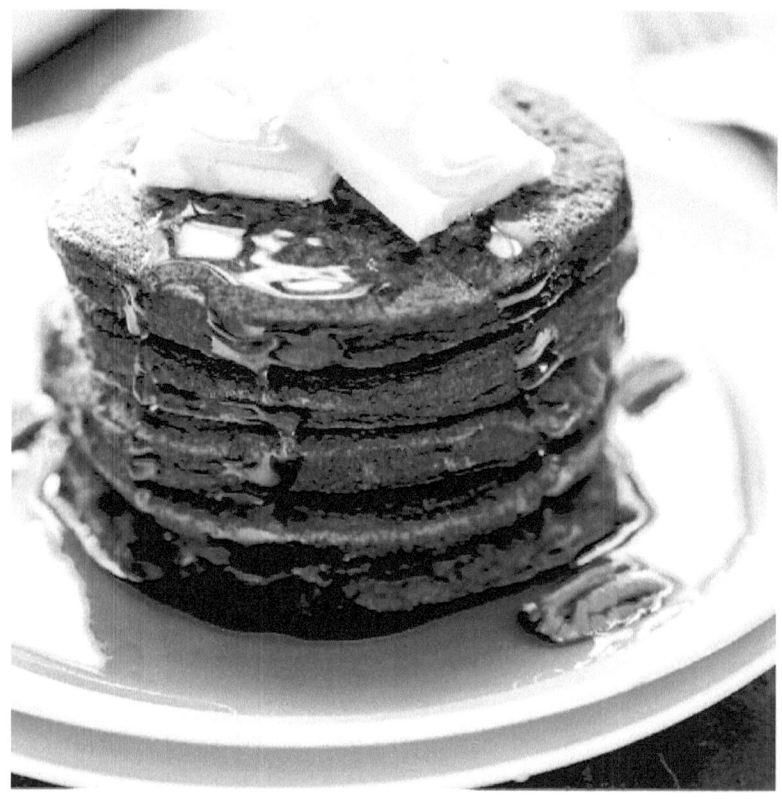

Serving: 4

Preparation Time: 5 Minutes

Cook Time: 15 Minutes

Total Time: 20 Minutes

Ingredients:

0.7 oz. (20 g) oats

three.2 oz. (92 g) liquid egg whites

1 oz. (28 g) pumpkin puree

1 scoop significant Proteins Collagen Peptides

½ tsp. Cinnamon

2 tsp. Stevia within the uncooked

Cooking spray

Sugar-free syrup (non-compulsory)

Apple (non-compulsory)

Directions:

1. Mix all of the constituents (besides the cooking spray) in a blender or Nutribullet and mixture except tender.

2. If you don't have a blender, use oat flour as a substitute of oats and mix it by way of hand.

3. Coat a small pan with cooking spray and placed on medium-high heat.

4. Pour a third of the batter into the pan, spreading it evenly.

5. Let the pancake cook dinner for about 2 minutes or except the sides of the pancake go light brown, earlier than flipping it over and cooking for two minutes on the opposite side.

6. Prepare dinner the opposite two pancakes the same method.

7. Serve with sugar-free syrup, apple pieces, and somewhat Stevia sprinkled on prime.

Low-Carb Cauliflower Oatmeal

Low-Carb Cauliflower Oatmeal is an mighty low-carb and grain-free alternative to natural oatmeal. It's simply as tasty and effortless to make however with lots fewer carbs and calories.

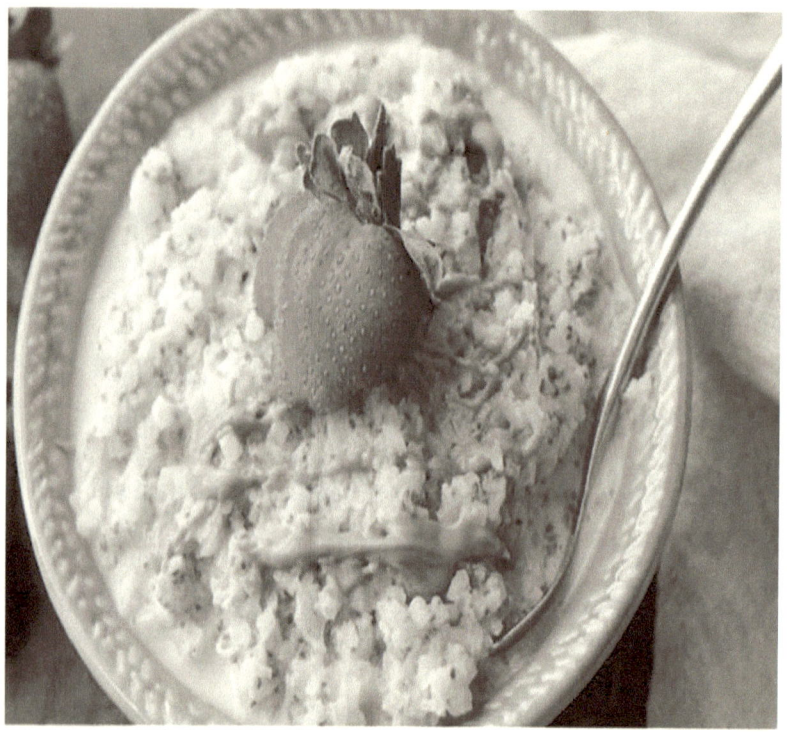

Serving: 2

Preparation Time: 5 Minutes

Cook Time: 15 Minutes

Total Time: 20 Minutes

Ingredients:

1 cup cauliflower rice

½ cup unsweetened almond milk

½ tsp. Cinnamon

¼ tsp Stevia

½ tbsp. Peanut butter

1 strawberry, sliced

Directions:

1. Location cauliflower rice in a pot with milk, cinnamon, and Stevia. Bring to a boil at the same time stirring.

2. Once boiling, scale back to a medium-low warmth and proceed stirring until favored thickness (~8-10 minutes).

3. If the combination becomes too thick, stir in additional milk to skinny it out.

4. Cast off from the warmness and transfer cauliflower oatmeal to a bowl.

5. Drizzle with creamy peanut butter and high with sliced strawberries.

Low Carb Cottage Cheese Pancakes

With these protein filled Low Carb Cottage Cheese Pancakes, you can enjoy America's favorite breakfast without the guilty conscience.

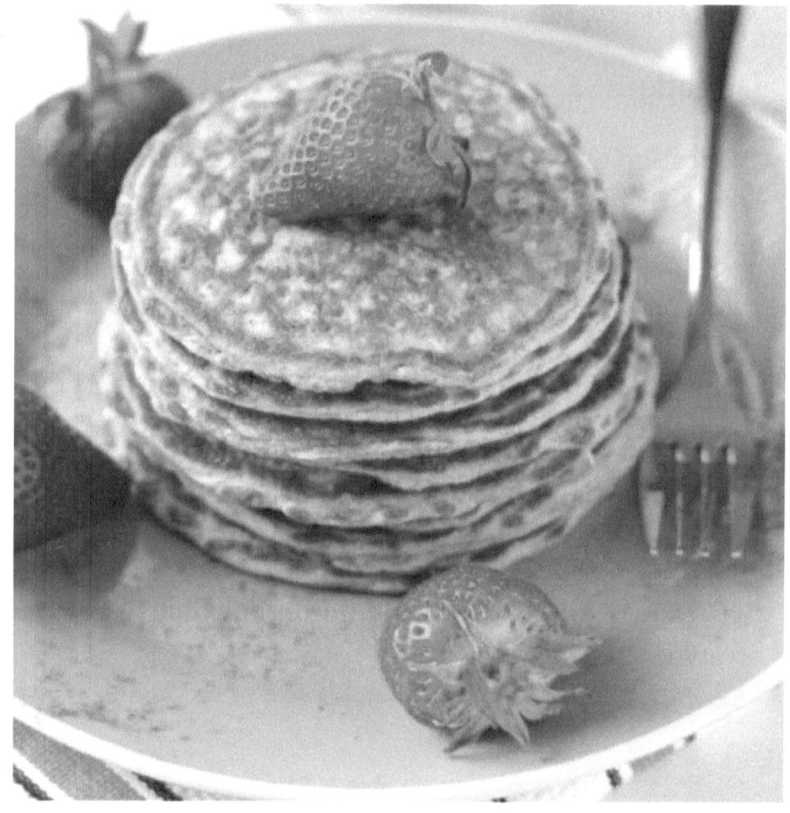

Serving: 4

Preparation Time: 5 Minutes

Cook Time: 10 Minutes

Total Time: 15 Minutes

Ingredients:

½ cup low-fat cottage cheese

¼ cup oats

? cup egg Whites (2 egg whites)

1 tsp. vanilla extract

1 tbsp. Stevia in the raw (only if you want the pancakes to be sweet)

Directions:

1. Pour cottage cheese and egg whites into the blender first, and then add oats, vanilla extract, and a little stevia.

2. Blend to a smooth consistency.

3. Put a pan with a little cooking spray on medium heat and fry each pancake until golden on both sides.

4. Present with peanut butter, berries or sugar-free jam.

10 Healthy Diabetic Lunch Ideas

Chicken and Egg Salad

This healthy bird and egg salad is one in every of my go-to lunch recipes. It tastes effective, is so easy to make you can barely call it cooking, and that you could make a enormous batch and store it within the fridge for days.

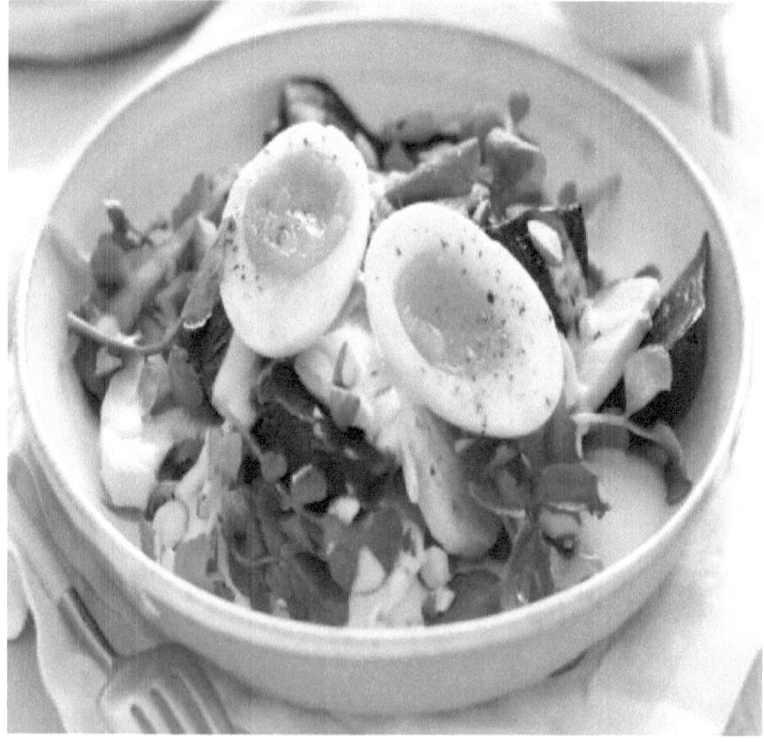

Serving: 5

Preparation Time: 5 Minutes

Cook Time: 10 Minutes

Total Time: 15 Minutes

Ingredients:

2 cooked fowl breasts

three difficult-boiled eggs

2 tbsp. Fats-free mayo

1 tbsp. Curry powder

Chives or basil (not obligatory)

Salt (optional)

Directions:

1. Bake the chook within the oven at 365 F (185 C) for roughly 20 min (assess with a knife that the chicken is cooked all of the manner via).

2. Boil the eggs for 8 minutes.

3. Reduce chicken and eggs into chew-sized portions.

4. Mix the mayo with curry powder (i love to use a number of curry powder. With half of a tablespoon and taste before including extra).

5. Combine everything in a enormous bowl and mix.

6. Let it cool within the fridge for at least 10 minutes (it gets even higher in the event you leave it in the fridge in a single day).

7. Serve on toast or cakes with chives and a bit of salt on high.

Tuna Nicoise Salad

A fresh tackle the traditional Tuna Nicoise Salad with a moderately spicy parsley and mustard dressing.

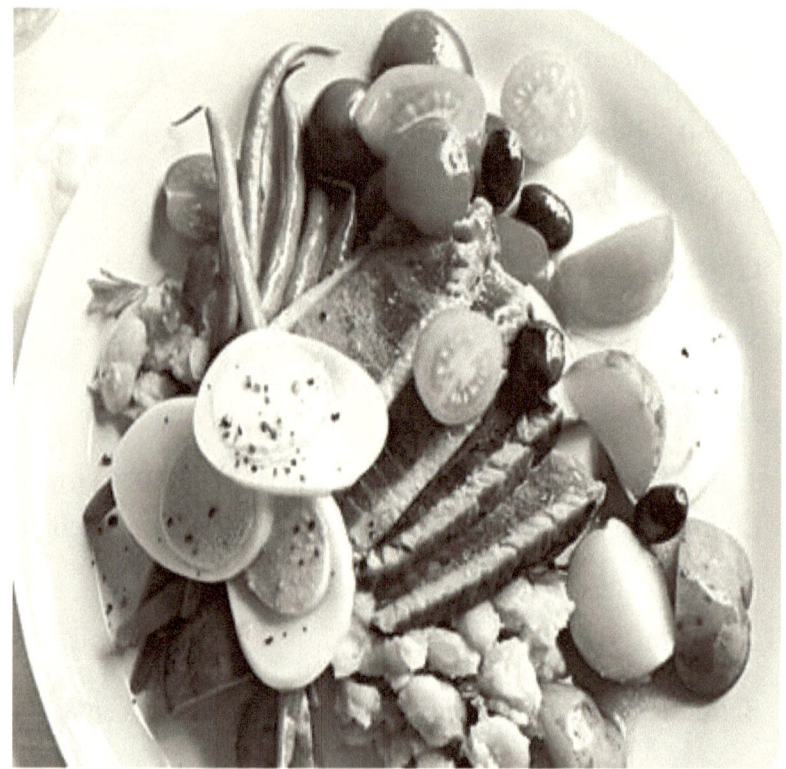

Serving: 4

Preparation Time: 5 Minutes

Cook Time: 10 Minutes

Total Time: 15 Minutes

Ingredients:

4 oz. Ahi tuna steak

1 entire egg

3 oz. Baby spinach (2 cups)

2 oz. Inexperienced beans

1½ oz. Broccoli

½ purple bell pepper

3½ oz. Cucumber

1 radish

3 large black olives

Handful of parsley

1 tsp. Olive oil

1 tsp. Balsamic vinegar

½ tsp. Dijon mustard

½ tsp. Pepper

Directions:

1. Boil the egg and set it aside to chill.

2. Steam broccoli and beans and put aside (2-3 minutes in the microwave with a little bit water does the trick or three minutes in a pot of boiling water).

3. Season the tuna with pepper on either side and cook it in a pan with a little bit oil on high warmth for 2 minutes on every facet.

4. Put the cleaned spinach into the bowl or plate you need to serve the salad in.

5. Reduce bell pepper, cucumber, and egg into dice-sized portions and add to the spinach.

6. Reduce the radish into slices and add along side the broccoli, beans, and olives.

7. Slice the tuna and add to the salad.

8. Whisk together olive oil, balsamic vinegar, mustard, salt, and pepper.

9. Chop the parsley and add it to the vinaigrette.

10. Use a spoon to drizzle the vinaigrette over the salad or use it as a dipping sauce.

Spinach Rolls

This is my favorite vegetarian recipe! It's easy, savory, and filling. Super yummy!

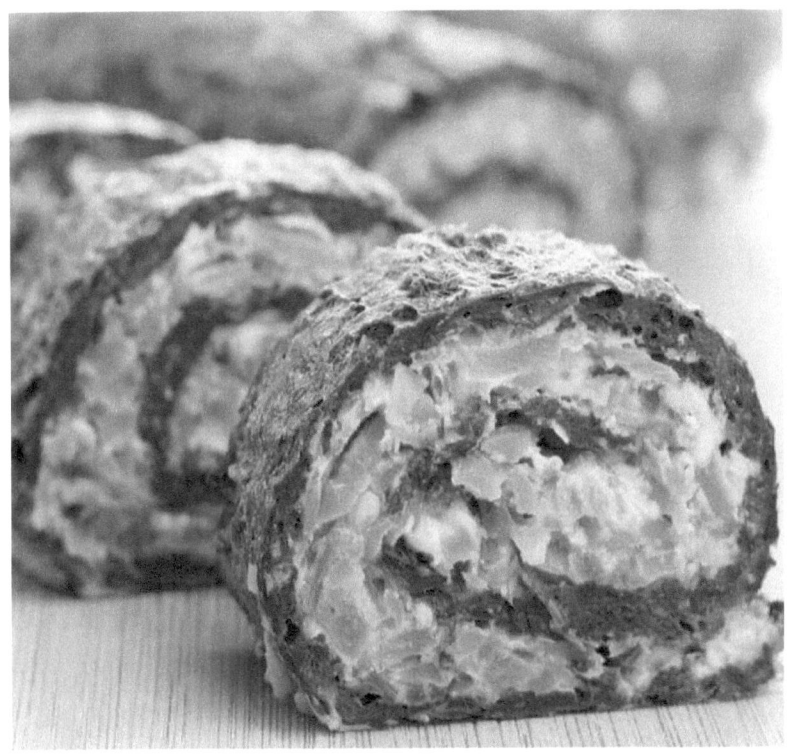

Serving: 3

Preparation Time: 10 Minutes

Cook Time: 50 Minutes

Total Time: 1 Hour

Ingredients:

16 oz. Frozen spinach leaves

3 eggs

2½ oz. Onion

2 oz. Carrot

1 oz. Little-fat mozzarella cheese

4 oz. Fats-free cottage cheese

¾ cup parsley

1 cloves garlic

1 tsp. Curry powder

¼ tsp. Chili flakes

1 tsp. Salt

1 tsp. Pepper

Cooking spray

Directions:

1. Preheat oven to four hundred° F (200° C).

2. Thaw the spinach and squeeze out the water (you need to use a strainer). To speed up the thawing method, that you would be able to microwave the spinach for a couple of minutes.

3. Mix spinach, 2 eggs, mozzarella, garlic, 1/2 the salt, and pepper in a mixing bowl.

4. Situation parchment paper on a baking sheet and spray with cooking spray. Transfer the spinach combination to the sheet

and press it flat, about 10x12 inches in size and roughly ½ an inch thick.

5. Heat for almost half hour. When done, put aside to chill on a rack. It'll get the feel/seem of a rather thick seaweed mat (when you ever have sushi, what I'm speaking about).

6. Don't turn off the oven! You'll need it again in just a little.

7. Finely slice onion and parsley. Grate the carrots.

8. Fry the onions for roughly a minute in a skillet with a bit of cooking spray. Add carrots and parsley to the pan and let it simmer for about 2 min.

9. Add cottage cheese, curry, chili, the opposite half of the salt, and pepper and mix in brief.

10. Remove the skillet off the heat and include an egg.

11. Combine all of it collectively and unfold the filling over the now cool spinach mat.

12. Don't unfold it all of the solution to the corners, or it's going to spill out whilst you roll it up.

13. Cautiously roll up the spinach mat and filling. Bake for 25 minutes.

14. Take out the roll and let it cool for five-10 min earlier than reducing it into slices and serving.

Healthy Turkey Meatballs (Without Breadcrumbs)

These Healthy Turkey Meatballs without Breadcrumbs are juicy little protein bombs packed with flavor.

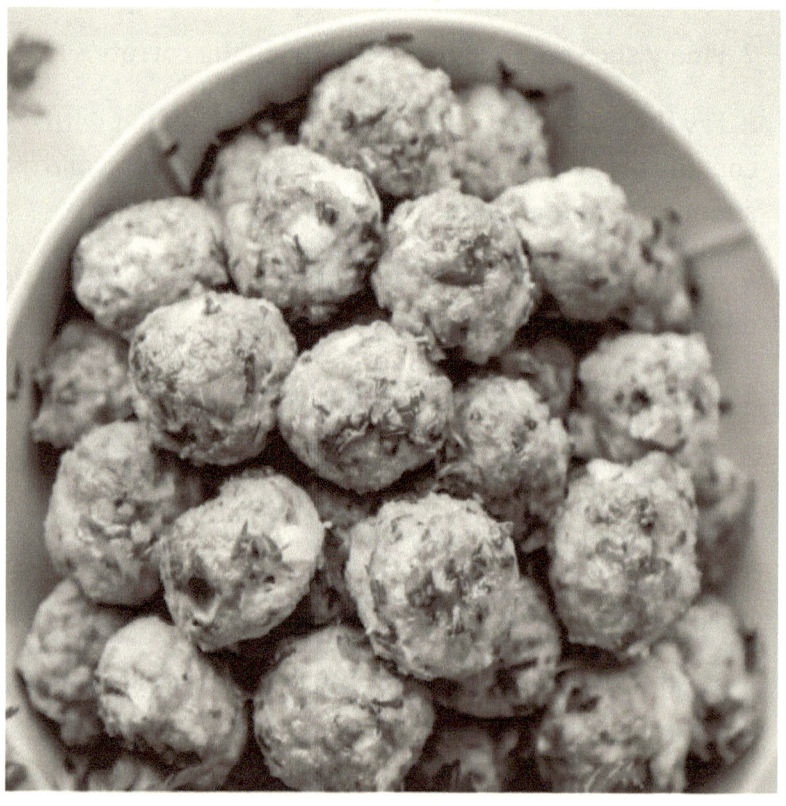

Serving: 6

Preparation Time: 5 Minutes

Cook Time: 50 Minutes

Total Time: 55 Minutes

Ingredients:

20 ounces. ground turkey

3.5 troy. present day or solidified spinach

¼ container oats

2 egg whites

2 celery sticks

3 cloves garlic

½ unpracticed chime pepper

½ purple onion

½ container parsley

½ tsp. Cumin

1 tsp. Mustard powder

1 tsp. Thyme

½ tsp. Turmeric

½ tsp. Chipotle pepper

1 tsp. Salt

Squeeze of pepper

Directions:

1. Preheat the stove to 350 F (175 C)

2. Hack onion, garlic, and celery in all respects finely (or utilize a dinners processor) and situated it in a major mixing bowl

3. Transfer turkey, egg whites, oats, and flavors to the bowl and mix totally. Ensure there are no pockets of flavors or oats inside the blend

4. Hack spinach, green peppers (simple out the stem and seeds first) and parsley. The segments ought to be the extent of a dime

5. Transfer the vegetables to the bowl and combine every last bit of it

6. Line a preparing sheet with material paper

7. Fold the turkey mix into 15 balls (roughly the size of hitting the fairway balls) and circumstance them on the heating sheet

8. Prepare for 25 minutes, aside from cooked through

Healthy Curried Chicken Salad With Apples

This healthful Curry bird Salad with Apples is a fit (and tastier) low-fat variation of the traditional fowl salad.

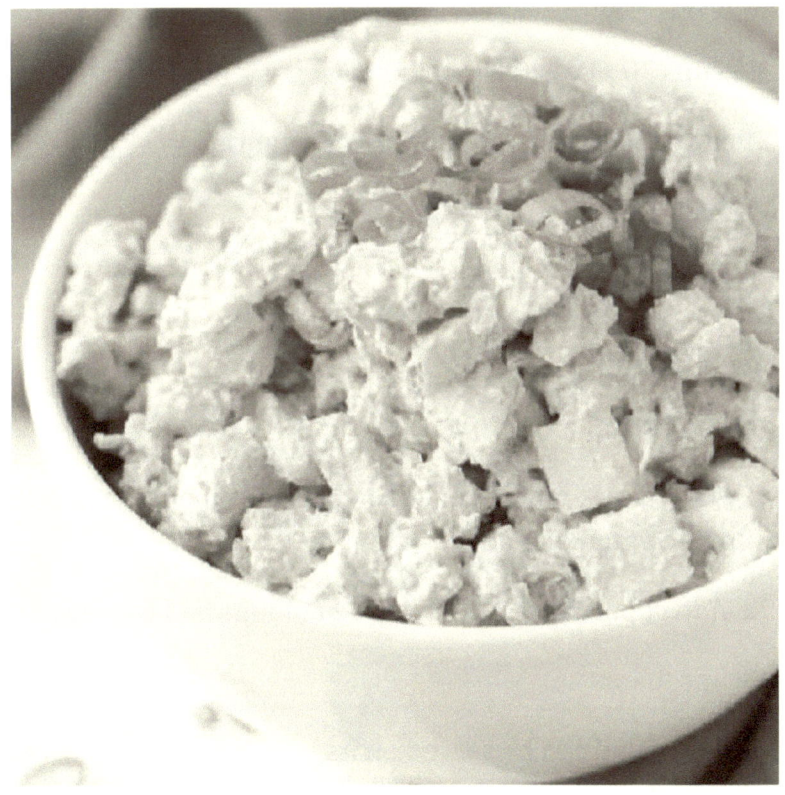

Serving: 7

Preparation Time: 5 Minutes

Cook Time: 15 Minutes

Total Time: 20 Minutes

Ingredients:

1 lbs. (450 g) cooked chicken breast, diced

1 Granny Smith apple, diced

2 celery stalks, diced

2 inexperienced onions, diced

½ cup (70 g) cashews, chopped

1 cup (280 g) non-fat plain Greek yogurt

1 tbsp. Tahini

Four tsp. Curry powder

1 tsp. Ground cinnamon

Directions:

1. Mix yogurt, tahini, curry powder and cinnamon in a significant mixing bowl

2. Add chook, apple, celery, green onions and cashews.

3. Stir to mix

4. This salad can be served on its possess, as a sandwich, or in a scooped out papaya to give it much more of a tropical think

Healthy Homemade Chicken Nuggets

These healthful do-it-yourself hen Nuggets taste so first-class you gained't consider they're truly excellent for you! They're low-carb, grain-free, and incorporate only six elements.

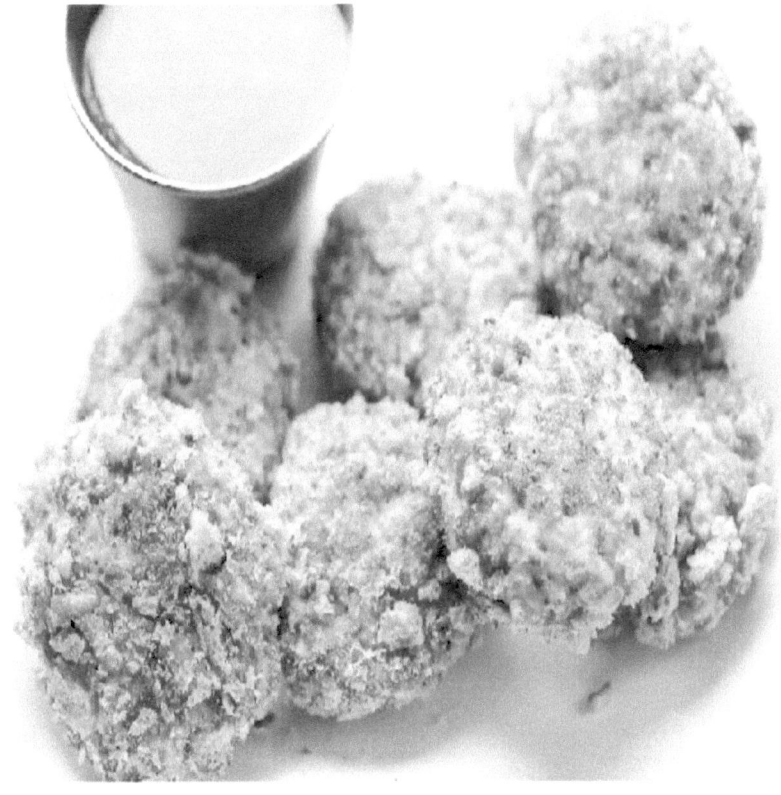

Serving: 3

Preparation Time: 5 Minutes

Cook Time: 45 Minutes

Total Time: 50 Minutes

Ingredients:

2 chook breasts, boneless and skinless

½ cup almond flour

1 tbsp. Italian seasoning

2 tbsp. extra virgin olive oil

½ tsp. Salt

½ tsp. Pepper

Directions:

1. Preheat oven to four hundred F (200 C). Put together a enormous baking sheet with parchment paper.

2. In a bowl, stir together the almond flour, Italian seasoning, salt, and pepper.

3. Reduce any ultimate fats off the fowl breasts and discard. Then slice into 1-inch thick pieces.

4. Spray the bird slices with the extra virgin olive oil.

5. Location each piece into the bowl with the flour and cover liberally. You can then Move to the prepared heating sheet.

6. Bake for 20 minutes, then flip the broiler on and situation below the broiler 3-four minutes to make the outside crispy.

7. Serve immediately with mustard or hot sauce.

Beef Fajitas You Can Make in 15 Minutes

You can make this easy fajita recipe in only 15 min. to get a delicious and healthy high-protein dinner.

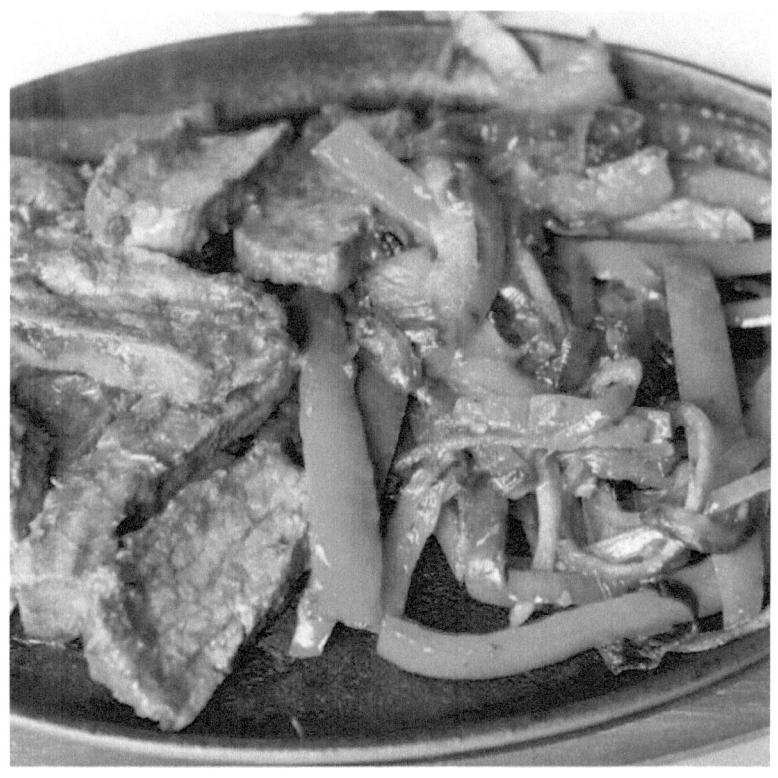

Serving: 6

Preparation Time: 5 Minutes

Cook Time: 15 Minutes

Total Time: 20 Minutes

Ingredients:

1 lbs. Red meat stir-fry strips

1 medium crimson onion

1 crimson bell pepper

1 yellow bell pepper

½ tsp. Cumin

½ tsp. Chilli powder

Splash of oil

Salt

Pepper

Juice of half of a lime

Freshly chopped cilantro (also called coriander)

1 avocado

Directions:

1. Warmness a forged-iron skillet over medium warmth

2. Wash and deseed bell peppers and slice them into 1/4" (zero.5 cm) thick long stripes. Place it somewhere

3. Peel and slice purple onion. Place it somewhere

four. As soon as skillet is sizzling, add a splash of oil. When the oil is sizzling, add stir-fry strips in 2-three batches.

5. Make sure the strips do not touch each other. Salt and pepper each and every batch generously within the pan

6. Cook for roughly 1 minute per part, then eliminate and put aside on a plate and canopy to maintain warm

7. Include sliced onions and bell peppers to the Waiting meat juice. Season with cumin and chili powder and stir-fry unless desired consistency. (i love them nonetheless crunchy, so I most effective stir-fry for approximately 5 minutes should you like your greens softer, stir-fry for slightly longer).

8. Serve on a plate with sliced avocado, a drizzle of lemon juice, and a sprinkle of contemporary coriander.

Keto Cobb Salad

Keto Cobb Salad is an easy-to-make keto salad recipe that's low in carbs and filled with taste. Each serving comprises handiest 6 grams of internet carbs!

Serving: 2

Preparation Time: 5 Minutes

Cook Time: 5 Minutes

Total Time: 10 Minutes

Ingredients:

4 cherry tomatoes

½ avocado

1 hardboiled egg

2 cups mixed inexperienced salad

2 oz. Bird breast, shredded

1 oz. Feta cheese, crumbled

¼ cup cooked 1st Baron Verulam, crumbled

Directions:

1. Dice the tomatoes and avocado, and slice the hardboiled egg.

2. Place the combined inexperienced salad right into a colossal salad bowl or plate.

3. Measure out the shredded fowl breast, feta cheese, and crumbled Baron Verulam.

4. Place tomatoes, avocado, egg, bird, feta, and Francis Bacon in horizontal rows on prime of the veggies.

5. Non-compulsory: which you could add 1 tbsp. Of Ranch dressing for 73 calories and about eight grams of fats (not incorporated in nutrition information under).

6. Enjoy the entire serving.

Instant Pot Chicken Chili

This instant Pot fowl Chili is an effortless inexperienced chili (chile verde) without beans without problems made in the on the spot Pot!

Serving: 10

Preparation Time: 5 Minutes

Cook Time: 25 Minutes

Total Time: 30 Minutes

Ingredients:

1 tbsp. Vegetable oil

1 yellow onion, diced

four cloves garlic, minced

1 tsp. Floor cumin

1 tsp. Oregano

2½ lbs. Chook breasts, boneless & skinless

16 oz. Salsa verde

Toppings

2 packages queso fresco , crumbled (or bitter cream)

2 avocados, diced

8 radishes, chopped exceptional

Eight springs cilantro (not obligatory)

Directions:

1. Set the on the spot Pot to the sauté atmosphere, medium.

2. Add the vegetable oil.

3. Add the onion and cook for 3 minutes, stirring as a rule unless the onion starts offevolved to soften.

4. Add the garlic, and stir for an extra minute.

5. Add the cumin and oregano and stir for another minute.

6. Pour ½ of the salsa verde into the pot. Prime with the chook breasts and pour the final salsa verde over the chicken.

7. Position the lid on the immediate Pot and set to "guide". Set the stopwatch for 10 minutes.

8. Use a common release (let the on the spot Pot liberate the strain through itself).

9. Do away with the bird from the pot and shred the chook with a fork.

10. Return the chook to the pot and stir to mix.

11. Serve in a bowl with the toppings or use for tacos.

12. Additional instantaneous Pot chook Chili will also be frozen in an airtight container.

Smoked Salmon and Cream Cheese Wraps

Smoked salmon and cream cheese must be some of the iconic breakfast/brunch combinations. The flavors of punchy smoked salmon and delicate cream cheese match perfectly with the sharp onion and fragrant herbs in these Smoked Salmon and Cream Cheese Wraps.

Serving: 2

Preparation Time: 5 Minutes

Cook Time: 15 Minutes

Total Time: 20 Minutes

Ingredients:

1 eight-inch low carb flour tortilla

2 oz. Smoked salmon

2 tsp. Low fat cream cheese

1¼ oz. Purple onion

Handful arugula

½ tsp. Fresh or dried basil

Pinch of pepper

Directions:

1. Heat the tortilla within the oven or microwave (pro tip: warm it between 2 portions of moist paper towel to hold it from drying out).

2. Combine cream cheese, basil, and pepper, and spread it onto the tortilla.

3. Prime it off with the salmon, arugula, and finely sliced onion.

4. Roll up the wrap and enjoy!

10 Healthy Dinner Recipes for Diabetics

Healthy Stuffed Chicken Breast

I could eat this stuffed hen breast every day. Its super tender, tastes extraordinary, and is a healthful meal all by way of itself – no facets required!

Serving: 4

Preparation Time: 5 Minutes

Cook Time: 25 Minutes

Total Time: 30 Minutes

Ingredients:

1 fowl breast

1 oz. Low-fats mozzarella

1 artichoke coronary heart (from a can)

1 tsp. tomato, sliced

5 huge basil leaves

1 clove garlic

¼ tsp. Curry powder

¼ tsp. Paprika

Pinch of pepper

Toothpicks

Directions:

1. Preheat the oven to 365 F (185 C).

2. Cut the hen breast practically halfway via with a sharp knife.

3. Chop up the mozzarella, artichoke, basil, tomato, and garlic. Mix to combine and stuff it into the cut fowl breast.

4. Use a number of toothpicks to shut the bird breast across the stuffing (you can find how in the video above).

5. Location the chicken breast on a baking sheet or aluminum foil, and season it with pepper, curry powder, and paprika.

6. Bake for round 20 minutes (relying on the scale of the fowl breast).

7. Take into account to do away with the toothpicks before serving, and you're done!

8. Not obligatory: To make the chicken breast much more smooth, begin by means of brining it in salt water as described in my put up "easy methods to prepare dinner The excellent hen Breast".

Low Carb Zucchini Lasagna

This Low Carb Zucchini Lasagna is a healthful and tasty alternative to traditional lasagna. You don't need pasta or a heavy sauce for this scrumptious lasagna!

Serving: 5

Preparation Time: 20 Minutes

Cook Time: 1 Hour, 20 Minutes

Total Time: 1 Hour, 40 Minutes

Ingredients:

16 oz. Floor red meat, ninety two%

2 medium zucchini

4½ oz. Onion

2 cloves garlic

1 serrano chili

3 tomatoes

5½ oz. Mushrooms

½ cube Knorr chook bouillon

½ cup shredded low-fats mozzarella

1 tsp. Paprika

1 tsp. Dried thyme

1 tsp. Dried basil

Salt & pepper

Cooking spray

Directions:

1. Use a julienne peeler to reduce the zucchini into ½-inch (1 cm) slices. Sprinkle lightly with salt and set aside for 10 minutes.

2. Blot the zucchini slices with a paper towel and grill or broil them within the oven for three minutes at high warmth.

3. after broiling, location the zucchini on paper towels (you wish to have to get as so much of the liquid out as feasible).

4. Reduce off the ends of the tomatoes and make an X insertion on top. Locate boiling water for a couple of minutes. Pour cold water over, and peel off the skin.

5. Roughly chop onions, garlic, chili, peeled tomatoes, and mushrooms.

6. Add a little cooking spray to a deep skillet and fry the garlic, onion and chili for 1 min.

7. Add the tomatoes and mushrooms to the skillet and sauté the vegetables for yet another 4 minutes. Then take them off the heat and set aside.

8. Cook the meat in the equal skillet with the paprika except entirely browned.

9. Add the vegetables back into the skillet together with the chook bouillon and last spices and let it simmer for 25 minutes over low warmness.

10. Warmness the oven to 375 degrees F (a hundred ninety C)

11. Line a small baking tray with parchment paper and use 1/3 of the zucchini to make a layer within the backside.

12. Put 1/3 of the meat sauce on prime. Add yet another layer of zucchini and continue like this except you're out of sauce and zucchini

13. Unfold shredded mozzarella on top and bake for 35 minutes

14. Take the lasagna out of the oven and enable to relaxation for 10 minutes before serving.

Spinach Rolls

That is my favorite vegetarian recipe! It's convenient, savory, and filling. Super yummy.

Serving: 4

Preparation Time: 5 Minutes

Cook Time: 55 Minutes

Total Time: 1 Hour

Ingredients:

16 oz. Frozen spinach leaves

3 eggs

2½ oz. Onion

2 oz. Carrot

1 oz. Low-fats mozzarella cheese

four oz. cottage cheese

¾ cup parsley

1 cloves garlic

1 tsp. Curry powder

¼ tsp. Chili flakes

1 tsp. Salt

1 tsp. Pepper

Cooking spray

Directions:

1. Preheat oven to four hundred° F (200° C).

2. Thaw the spinach and squeeze out the water (you need to use a strainer). To speed up the thawing approach, that you could microwave the spinach for a couple of minutes.

3. Combine spinach, 2 eggs, mozzarella, garlic, half of the salt, and pepper in a mixing bowl.

4. Position parchment paper on a baking sheet and spray with cooking spray. Move the spinach combination to the sheet and press it flat, about 10x12 inches in measurement and roughly ½ an inch thick.

5. Heat for almost half-hour. When carried out, put aside to cool on a rack. It's going to get the texture/look of a relatively thick seaweed mat (if you ever have sushi, you realize what I'm speaking about). Don't turn off the oven! You'll want it once more in a little bit.

6. Sliced parsley and onion. Grate the carrots.

7. Fry the onions for roughly a minute in a skillet with a little bit cooking spray. Add carrots and parsley to the pan and let it simmer for roughly 2 min. Add cottage cheese, curry, chili, the other 1/2 of the salt, and pepper and blend in brief.

8. Take the skillet off the warmth and add an egg. Combine it all collectively and unfold the filling over the now cool spinach mat. Don't spread it all of the method to the corners, or it's going to spill out while you roll it up.

9. Cautiously roll up the spinach mat and filling. Heat for about 25 minutes.

10. Take out the roll and let it cool for 5-10 min earlier than cutting it into slices and serving.

Coconut Chicken Soup

The wealthy coconut aroma of this handy Coconut chicken Soup will warm your stomach and soul! Loaded with many specific veggies and lean chook breast, this soup will hold you full and satisfied for a very long time.

Serving: 8

Preparation Time: 5 Minutes

Cook Time: 55 Minutes

Total Time: 1 Hour

Ingredients:

1 lb. Fowl breast, thinly sliced

Salt & pepper, to taste

1 tbsp. Coconut oil (or vegetable oil)

1 small onion, thinly sliced into 1/2 moons

2 garlic cloves, minced

1 inch piece ginger, peeled and minced

1 medium zucchini, reduce into quarters lengthwise and diced

0.80 lb. Pumpkin, cubed into ½ inch portions (1 cup),

1 crimson bell pepper, seeds eliminated and thinly sliced

1 small chili or jalapeño pepper, seeds removed and thinly sliced

14 oz. Lite coconut milk (1 can)

2 cups hen broth

Juice of 1 lime

Handful cilantro leaves (not obligatory)

Directions:

1. Season the sliced chicken breast generously with salt and pepper.

2. in a giant (5-6 quart) soup pot, heat the coconut oil over excessive warmth and add the bird breast. Stir-fry over high warmness for 4-5 minutes, or unless the chook is no longer red on the external.

3. Add the sliced onion, minced garlic, and minced ginger and proceed to stir-fry for an additional 2-3 minutes.

4. Include the cubed pumpkin and diced zucchini, and mix. Add the sliced bell pepper, sliced chili or jalapeño pepper, coconut milk, chicken broth, and lime juice. Stir the whole lot together.

5. Bring to a boil, then minimize the warmness, duvet, and allow to simmer for approximately 20 minutes, or until the pumpkin is wholly cooked.

6. Season with additional salt and pepper, if favored. Garnish with cilantro leaves to serve.

Marinated Turkey Breast

This marinated turkey breast needs to be certainly one of my favourite recipes for a fast, healthy meal. It combines highest taste with minimum work within the kitchen.

Serving: 8

Preparation Time: 5 Minutes

Cook Time: 55 Minutes

Total Time: 1 Hour

Ingredients:

4 oz. Turkey breast

1 tsp. Olive oil

1½ tsp. Balsamic vinegar

¼ tsp. Garlic powder

¼ tsp. Dried basil

¼ tsp. Thyme

¼ tsp. Pepper

Directions:

1. Mix basil, thyme, garlic powder, and pepper with balsamic vinegar and olive oil in a bowl or colossal Ziploc.

2. Reduce the turkey breast into thumb-sized portions or strips and location in the marinade for at least 20-30 minutes.

3. Remove the turkey from marinade and fry in a skillet for 5-8 minutes at medium warmness (relying on the scale of the turkey strips. Turkey must be entirely cooked).

Healthy & Easy Beef Fajitas You Can Make in 15 Minutes

You could make this convenient fajita recipe in simplest 15 min. To get a delicious and healthy excessive-protein dinner

Serving: 6

Preparation Time: 5 Minutes

Cook Time: 15 Minutes

Total Time: 20 Minutes

Ingredients:

1 lbs. hamburger sautéed food strips

1 medium pink onion

1 blood red ringer pepper

1 yellow ringer pepper

½ tsp. cumin

½ tsp. bean stew powder

sprinkle of oil

Salt

Pepper

Juice of 1/2 a lime

Naturally cleaved cilantro (likewise alluded to as coriander)

1 avocado

Directions:

1. Warmness a skillet in medium

2. Wash and deseed ringer peppers and cut them into 1/4" (0.five cm) thick long stripes.

3. Strip and cut purple onion. Set apart when skillet is warm, include a sprinkle of oil. While the oil is warm, include pan fried food strips in 2-3 clusters.

4. Guarantee the strips don't contact each extraordinary. Salt and pepper each clump liberally in the container

5. get ready supper for around 1 moment as indicated by feature, at that point expel and set apart on a plate and spread to look after warmth

6. Include cut onions and chime peppers to the rest of the meat juice. Season with cumin and bean stew powder and pan fried food till wanted consistency. (I adore them in any case crunchy, so I just pan fried food for around five minutes.

7. On the off chance that you need your veggies gentler, pan sear for somewhat more).

8. Serve on a plate with cut avocado, a shower of lemon juice, and a sprinkle of shimmering coriander.

Prosciutto Wrapped Chicken Breast with Cream Cheese

Hen Breast Wrapped in Cream Cheese and Prosciutto is an amazingly handy and healthy method to bake the best juicy and delicious fowl breast.

Serving: 2

Preparation Time: 5 Minutes

Cook Time: 35 Minutes

Total Time: 40 Minutes

Ingredients:

1 chook breast

1.Four oz. Finely sliced prosciutto (Parma ham)

1.3 oz. Cream cheese (low-fat)

5-10 fresh basil leaves (depending on dimension)

Pepper

Directions:

1. Location the prosciutto slices on a bit of aluminum foil so the edges overlap fairly.

2. Unfold the cream cheese evenly onto the prosciutto. Pro TIP: Take the cream cheese out of the fridge quarter-hour earlier than you start utilizing it to let it warm up a bit of. In order to make it so much less complicated to work with.

3. Position the fresh basil leaves on top so they cover the cream cheese.

4. Gently, wrap the prosciutto, cream cheese, and basil leaves across the hen breast and grind a bit of pepper on top (or a lot of pepper if you're like me and love pepper).

5. Bake the Prosciutto Wrapped hen Breast with Cream Cheese within the oven for 25-half-hour (depending on how giant the bird breast is) at 380 F (a hundred ninety C).

6. Let the chicken relaxation for a minute external the over before slicing and serving. Revel in!

Baked Boneless Pork Chops in Tomato Sauce

Baked Boneless Pork Chops in Tomato Sauce is a excessive-protein recipe you'll to find yourself making again and again. These pork chops are juicy, delicate, and stuffed with taste!

Serving: 5

Preparation Time: 5 Minutes

Cook Time: 35 Minutes

Total Time: 40 Minutes

Ingredients:

4 Thick pork cleaves

1 little yellow onion

four cloves garlic

28 oz. Diced canned tomatoes (one huge can)

5 oz. Low-fat mozzarella

1 Knorr hen bouillon dice

1 tsp. Paprika

1 tsp. Dried oregano

Salt and pepper

Cooking splash

Directions:

1. Preheat stove to 400 F (200 C).

2. Slice onions. Strip and cut the garlic.

3. Cut the fats skin off the pork hacks (if necessary).

4. Coat a skillet with cooking splash. Season pork cleaves with pepper and burn for around 2 minutes on each side (except if delicate dark colored).

5. Take the pork slashes off the warmth and position them in a profound preparing container.

6. Add onion rings and garlic to the skillet you used to singe the pork cleaves and burn for around a moment on each side.

7. Include tomato, bouillon block, and flavors to the dish and mix everything all things considered.

8. Give it a chance to stew for 2 minutes after which pour over the pork slashes.

9. Sprinkle cheddar on prime and heat for 20 minutes.

10. Remove the pork cleaves from the stove and let them rest inside the search for gold minutes before serving.

Instant Pot Chicken Chili

This instantaneous Pot chicken Chili is an easy inexperienced chili (chile verde) without beans without difficulty made in the on the spot Pot!

Serving: 10

Preparation Time: 5 Minutes

Cook Time: 25 Minutes

Total Time: 30 Minutes

Ingredients:

1 tbsp. Vegetable oil

1 yellow onion, diced

four cloves garlic, minced

1 tsp. Ground cumin

1 tsp. Oregano

2½ lbs. Chook breasts, boneless & skinless

sixteen oz. Salsa verde

Toppings

2 applications queso fresco , crumbled (or bitter cream)

2 avocados, diced

8 radishes, chopped great

Eight springs cilantro (not obligatory)

Directions:

1. Set the instantaneous Pot to the sauté atmosphere, medium.

2. Add the vegetable oil.

3. Add the onion and cook for three minutes, stirring in most cases except the onion starts to melt.

4. Add the garlic, and stir for another minute.

5. Add the cumin and oregano and stir for a different minute.

6. Pour ½ of the salsa verde into the pot. High with the hen breasts and pour the remaining

7. Salsa verde over the chook.

8. Position the lid on the immediate Pot and set to "guide". Set the timer for 10 minutes.

9. Use a traditional liberate (let the immediate Pot unencumber the strain via itself). As soon as complete, put off the bird from the pot and shred the chook with a fork.

10. Return the fowl to the pot and stir to mix.

11. Serve in a bowl with the toppings or use for tacos.

12. Extra instantaneous Pot chook Chili will also be frozen in an hermetic container.

Healthy Turkey Meatballs (Without Breadcrumbs)

These healthful Turkey Meatballs without Breadcrumbs are juicy little protein bombs filled with taste.

Serving: 7

Preparation Time: 5 Minutes

Cook Time: 45 Minutes

Total Time: 50 Minutes

Ingredients:

20 oz. Floor turkey

3.5 oz. Recent or frozen spinach

¼ cup oats

2 egg whites

2 celery sticks

three cloves garlic

½ green bell pepper

½ red onion

½ cup parsley

½ tsp. Cumin

1 tsp. Mustard powder

1 tsp. Thyme

½ tsp. Turmeric

½ tsp. Chipotle pepper

1 tsp. Salt

Pinch of pepper

Directions:

1. Preheat the heating machine to 350 F (175 C)

2. Chop onion, garlic, and celery very finely (or use a meals processor) and put it in a colossal mixing bowl

3. Add turkey, egg whites, oats, and spices to the bowl and blend absolutely. Make sure there are no pockets of spices or oats within the mix

4. Chop spinach, inexperienced peppers (smooth out the stem and seeds first) and parsley. The portions will have to be the dimensions of a dime

5. Add the veggies to the bowl and blend all of it together

6. Line a heating pan with parchment paper

7. Roll the turkey blend into 15 balls (about the dimension of golf balls) and place them on the baking sheet

8. Bake for 25 minutes, unless cooked through

Lemon Chicken Piccata

Lemon chook Piccata is a finances-pleasant take on an Italian classic! Highly effortless and low carb, this piccata recipe is one you'll want to make over and over again!

Serving: 5

Preparation Time: 5 Minutes

Cook Time: 35 Minutes

Total Time: 40 Minutes

Ingredients:

2 skinless, boneless bird breasts

3 tbsp. Unsalted butter

1½ tbsp. All reason flour

¼ tsp. White pepper

¼ tsp. Salt

2 tbsp. Olive oil

? Cup dry white wine

? Cup low sodium chook inventory

¼ cup lemon juice

¼ cup drained capers

¼ cup Italian Parsley minced

Salt & pepper

Directions:

1. Slice every chook breasts in 1/2 lengthwise so you get 2 skinny bird slices from each and every breast (you will see that how they are supposed to seem within the 2d snapshot in this post).

2. If the chook slices are very thick, use a mallet or a further heavy object to flatten them fairly - you wish to have them not more than ½ inch (1.25 cm) thick.

3. Unfold the flour out thinly on a dinner plate. Add Pepper and Little salt.

4. Lightly dredge the fowl breast slices within the pro flour, shaking off extra flour. Place it where safe.

5. Heat a significant saute pan over medium-excessive heat. When the oil is shimmering, add the chook breast slices to the pan. Prepare dinner for three -four minutes except browned.

6. Turn the bird slices over and brown on the other part. Remove the hen slices from the pan and set aside.

7. Add the wine to the saute pan, stirring and scraping up the browned bits on the bottom of the pan.

8. Add the lemon juice and fowl stock. Develop the heat to high and boil until the sauce thickens - about 3 minutes.

9. Minimize the warmth to medium and add the butter.

10. Stir within the capers and parsley and add the hen breast slices again to the pan to rewarm.

11. Style the sauce and regulate the seasoning.

Serve!

10 Easy Low Carb Diabetic Desserts

Low-Carb Peanut Butter Cookies

These low-carb peanut butter cookies are a first-class healthy deal with, now not most effective are they delicious but additionally they are made in one bowl using simply 5 materials!

Serving: 10

Preparation Time: 10 Minutes

Cook Time: 20 Minutes

Total Time: 30 Minutes

Ingredients:

1 cup soft peanut butter no brought sugar

1 enormous egg

2/3 cup erythritol

half tsp. Baking soda

half tsp. Vanilla essence

Directions:

1. Preheat oven to 350F (one hundred eighty°C) and line a cookie tray with baking paper. Place it where safe

2. Add the erythritol to a Nutribullet or blender and blend until powdered. Place it somewhere safe.

3. Add all the components for the peanut butter cookies into a mixing bowl and mix unless a delicate dough varieties.

4. Range out 2 tbsp. Of the dough and roll between your arms to make circular balls and place for your cookie tray. Proceed except all the dough has been used.

5. Use a fork to press the cookies down and bake for 12 - quarter-hour relying in your oven.

6. As soon as they've cooked, remove from the oven and permit to cool for 25 minutes on the cookie tray. Do not touch them

7. Once they've cooled on the cookie tray, transfer the peanut butter cookies to a cooling rack and allow to chill for a further 15 minutes.

Chocolate Keto Fat Bombs

On the keto weight loss program and craving a chocolate treats? Look no extra than these Chocolate Keto fat Bombs.

Serving: 7

Preparation Time: 10 Minutes

Cook Time: 20 Minutes

Total Time: 30 Minutes

Ingredients:

¼ cup unsweetened Cacao (or Cocoa) powder

5 tbsp. Usual chunky peanut butter

6 tbsp. Hemp seeds, shelled

½ cup unrefined coconut oil

2 tbsp. Heavy cream

1 tsp. Vanilla extract

2 tbsp. Stevia

Directions:

1. Combine cocoa powder, peanut butter, and hemp seeds in a tremendous bowl.

2. Add room temperature coconut oil and mix until it becomes a paste.

3. Add cream, vanilla, and stevia and blend unless it turns into a paste once more.

Roll into balls.

4. You must be capable to make about 12 balls total, which equals 6 servings (2 balls = 1 serving).

5. Roll in shredded coconut (coconut integrated in diet information, but non-compulsory in case you are not a fan).

6. Place balls on parchment paper on a baking tray.

7. Freeze for 10 minutes or put within the fridge for a minimum of 30 minutes before serving.

8. Retailer within the freezer or fridge.

Low Carb Protein Cheesecake

I make this healthful low carb protein cheesecake to fulfill my cheesecake cravings without blowing a entire week's calorie budget. It's simple and scrumptious!

Serving: 5

Preparation Time: 5 Minutes

Cook Time: 1 Hour

Total Time: 1 Hour 5 Minutes

Ingredients:

8.5 oz. Low fats cottage cheese

2 egg whites

1 scoop vanilla protein powder

1 tbsp. Stevia

1 tsp. Vanilla extract

1 serving sugar-free Strawberry Jell-O

Water

Directions:

1. Preheat the oven to 325 F (one hundred sixty C).

2. Put together the Jell-O according to the instructional materials on the package and place in freezer.

3. Blend cottage cheese and egg whites unless the consistency is tender and with none lumps.

4. Pour the blend right into a bowl and whisk it together with the protein powder, Stevia, and vanilla extract.

5. Pour the mixture into a small nonstick pan and bake for 25 minutes.

6. Turn off the oven, leaving the cake in there while it cools down.

7. When the Jell-O is just about set (you will have to just be able to stir it), pour it over the cheesecake.

8. Let the cake set in the fridge for approximately 10-12 hours minimum earlier than enjoying.

Low Carb Chocolate Greek Yogurt Ice Cream

This scrumptious Low carb Chocolate Greek Yogurt Ice Cream is high in protein and low in calories. The ideal snack for a sizzling day or after a hard exercise.

Serving: 5

Preparation Time: 10 Minutes

Cook Time: 2 Hours

Total Time: 2 Hours, 10 Minutes

Ingredients:

2½ oz. Fat-free Greek yogurt

½ oz. Vanilla protein powder

1 tsp. Unsweetened cocoa powder

½ cup unsweetened almond milk

1 tsp. Vanilla extract

2 tbsp. Stevia to taste

Almonds & berries (not obligatory)

Directions:

1. Blend yogurt, protein powder, cocoa, stevia and almond milk absolutely.

2. In case you don't have a blender, this can be achieved by means of hand but requires a little work with a whisk.

3. Location in freezer or ice cream computing device.

4. In the event you don't have an ice cream computer (which we don't), take the ice cream out after an hour and switch it over gently with a spoon to avoid it fitting one giant ice block.

5. Do that once more each 30 min. Except it has the right consistency (it should take about 2hours total).

6. Which you can both eat it right away (after the two hours) or go away it within the freezer for up to every week.

7. Should you go away it within the freezer, take it out 5-10 min before you serve it to let it soften up a little bit.

8. Serve with almonds and fresh berries.

High-Protein Raspberry & Banana Mousse

High-Protein Raspberry & Banana Mousse is the perfect high protein snack! It has a thick silky consistency (like thick whipped cream) without any of the unhealthy ingredients you usually find in anything as good as this.

Serving: 5

Preparation Time: 5 Minutes

Cook Time: 15 Minutes

Total Time: 20 Minutes

Ingredients:

2 egg whites (ninety g liquid egg white)

1 tbsp. Stevia

2 oz. (60 g) frozen banana

1 ¾ oz. (45 g) frozen raspberry

contemporary berries (optional)

Directions:

1. Blend the egg whites and Stevia except the egg whites are organization (1-2 minutes).

2. You will have to be ready to preserve the blender the wrong way up without the egg whites falling out.

3. When the egg whites are firm, add the banana and berries and combination except the consistency is smooth and the whole lot is crimson.

4. Serve in a bowl with a couple of fresh berries or use as a side for my Cottage Cheese Pancakes.

Pumpkin Raspberry Muffins

These healthful raspberry pumpkin truffles taste so sinful that no person will consider that they are in reality low-carb, low-fats, and sugar-free when you tell them.

Serving: 10

Preparation Time: 10 Minutes

Cook Time: 30 Minutes

Total Time: 40 Minutes

Ingredients:

6.Three ozpumpkin

zero.5 cup coconut flour

four.5 Scoop vanilla protein powder

1 cup egg whites

1 cup frozen raspberries

1 cup Stevia within the uncooked

1 tsp. Cinnamon

½ tsp. Ginger

Cooking spray

Directions:

1. Preheat your oven to 375 F (a hundred ninety C)

2. Mix pumpkin and egg whites in a enormous bowl

3. Add all the last ingredients except the raspberries and mix good. Ensure no pockets of dry elements remain

4. Grease your muffin pan with slightly cooking spray

5. Crinkle the iced raspberries into the dough. You want to do this swiftly before the raspberries get delicate and lose their form

6. Scoop the dough into the pan. It should make 12 desserts

7. Bake the desserts for 15 min.

8. Take the desserts out of the oven and let them cool on a rack for minimal 10 min. Before serving

Strawberry Lemonade Popsicles (No Sugar Added)

Sweet, tart, and filled with strawberry goodness, these popsicles are a fresh, delightful treat sweetened simplest with a number of drops of stevia extract.

Serving: 8

Preparation Time: 10 Minutes

Cook Time: 30 Minutes

Total Time: 3 Hours, 10 Minutes

Ingredients:

¼ cup historical-customary oats

4 oz. Low fats cottage cheese

1½ lb. Strawberries

4 oz. Lemon juice, 4 lemons,

5 drops liquid Stevia

Directions:

1. Pulse oats in a high-powered blender or meals system except they turn into powder.

2. Add strawberries, cottage cheese, lemon juice, stevia, and pulse except delicate (if indispensable, discontinue the blender and push the components down with a spatula or the plunger that comes with the blender. Dont include any liquid!)

3. Pour the mixture into 6 popsicle molds and freeze until solid, at least three hours.

Keto Snickerdoodle Woopie Pies

Serving: 8

Preparation Time: 10 Minutes

Cook Time: 40 Minutes

Total Time: 50 Minutes

Ingredients:

For the Keto Snickerdoodles

3 Eggs, isolated

3 Tbsp Cream Cheddar

¼ Tsp Cream of Tartar

three Tbsp Granulated Sugar, partitioned (I utilized this one)

½ Tsp Cinnamon

For the Filling

½ Glass Cream Cheddar

¼ Glass Overwhelming Whipping Cream

1 Tbsp Sugar

1 Tsp Vanilla

½ Tsp Cinnamon

Directions:

1. for the Snickerdoodles

2. Preheat broiler to 300 F. Cautiously discrete the eggs. In a solitary bowl, join together the egg yolks, the cream cheddar and 1 tbsp of the sugar, aside from delicate.

3. In an extra bowl, add the cream of tartar to the egg whites, at that point beat on exorbitant speed with the exception of firm pinnacles type. This may progressively take a couple of minutes and will appear to be thick and not foamy.

4. At that point, cautiously overlap the egg yolk combo into the egg whites. Make an effort not to separate the cushiness of the egg whites.

5. Oil two heating sheets, at that point scoop the mix into 20 little adjusts.

6. Blend the rest of the sugar with the cinnamon, at that point sprinkle it onto everything about mists.

7. Bake for 30 minutes. Taking a gander at eagerly, as they consume viably. Let cool totally

8. For the Filling In a goliath bowl, beat the cream cheddar with the Sugar, until delicate. Gradually beat inside the vanilla, cinnamon and substantial cream.

9. Continue to beat the mix except if solid. Position inside the ice chest with the exception of the snickerdoodles cool.

10. When the snickerdoodles have cooled altogether, exchange the filling to a zipper lock pack. 11. Flip 1/2 of them topsy turvy. At that point cut the side of the ziplock, crush the filling equitably onto everything about. (utilize a spoon in the event

that you don't have any ziplocks) At that point duvet with the rest of.

12. Notice: retailer in an impermeable compartment inside the refrigerator.

Easy Chocolate Fudge Recipe (Vegan + Low Carb + Keto)

Serving: 8

Preparation Time: 10 Minutes

Cook Time: 2 Hours

Total Time: 2 Hours, 10 Minutes

Ingredients:

1 1/2 cups coconut butter

1 (13.sixty six fl oz) can complete-fats coconut milk

10 ounces bittersweet chocolate chips

Elective: flaked or coarse sea salt for topping

Directions:

1. Line an 8x8 inch baking pan with wax paper or foil.

2. In a small saucepan over low warmth, soften the coconut butter.

3. Stir in the coconut milk and chocolate chips.

4. Prepare dinner over low warm temperature, stirring more regularly than not, until the chocolate chips are melted.

5. pour the combination into the pan. optional: sprinkled flaked or coarse sea salt over the top.

6. Region in refrigerator unless set, approximately 2 hours. Slice before serving

Keto Brownies

These decadent keto truffles are insanely scrumptious, crispy across the edges and flawlessly gooey within the middle. They're so wealthy that just a few bites is all you must get your chocolate repair.

Serving: 10

Preparation Time: 10 Minutes

Cook Time: 40 Minutes

Total Time: 50 Minutes

Ingredients:

half of cup + 2 tablespoons salted butter, melted

1 cup granular swerve sweetener

2 massive eggs

2 teaspoons vanilla extract

half of cup lily's chocolate chips, melted

2 tablespoons coconut flour

2 tablespoons unsweetened cocoa powder

half teaspoons salt

half cup lily's chocolate chips

Directions:

1. Pre-warmth the oven to 350f and line a 8x8 steel baking pan with parchment paper. Drizzle the sheet with cooking spray.

2. Whisk the melted butter and the swerve collectively in a big mixing bowl till easy. Add eggs and vanilla and beat with an electric powered mixer for 1 minute.

3. add in the melted chocolate chips and stir till simply mixed. With a rubber spatula, add in the coconut flour, cocoa powder, salt, and stir till simply blended.

4. Crinkle inside the chocolate chips.

5. Pour the batter into the prepared pan and clean out the top with a spatula.

6. Bake within the oven for half-hour. eliminate from the oven and permit cool inside the pan for half-hour.

7. Cast off from the pan and reduce into 9 squares.

8. Keep in an airtight field.

12 Healthy diabetic chicken recipes

Healthy Stuffed Chicken Breast

I would eat this stuffed hen breast day by day. Its super tender, tastes super, and is a healthy meal all with the aid of itself – no aspects required!

Serving: 2

Preparation Time: 10 Minutes

Cook Time: 20 Minutes

Total Time: 30 Minutes

Ingredients:

1 chook breast

1 oz. Low-fat mozzarella

1 artichoke heart (from a can)

1 tsp. slash sundried tomato

5 big basil leaves

1 clove garlic

¼ tsp. Curry powder

¼ tsp. Paprika

Pinch of pepper

Toothpicks

Directions:

1. Preheat the oven to 365 F (185 C).

2. Cut the chook breast practically midway via with a pointy knife.

3. Chop up the mozzarella, artichoke, basil, tomato, and garlic. Mix to combine and stuff it into the reduce hen breast.

4. Use a couple of toothpicks to shut the hen breast across the stuffing (you will see how within the video above).

5. Position the fowl breast on a baking sheet or aluminum foil, and season it with pepper, curry powder, and paprika.

6. Bake for around 20 minutes (depending on the dimensions of the hen breast).

7. Recall to cast off the toothpicks before serving, and you are carried out!

8. Non-compulsory: To make the hen breast even more delicate, start by brining it in salt water as described in my post "tips on how to cook dinner The perfect bird Breast".

Coconut Chicken Soup

The rich coconut aroma of this handy Coconut fowl Soup will heat your stomach and soul! Loaded with many exclusive greens and lean fowl breast, this soup will hold you full and satisfied for a long time.

Serving: 5

Preparation Time: 10 Minutes

Cook Time: 45 Minutes

Total Time: 55 Minutes

Ingredients:

1 lb. Chicken breast, thinly sliced

Salt & pepper, to style

1 tbsp. Coconut oil (or vegetable oil)

1 small onion, thinly sliced into 1/2 moons

2 garlic cloves, minced

1 inch piece ginger, peeled and minced

1 medium zucchini, cut into quarters lengthwise and diced

zero.75 lb. Pumpkin, cubed into ½ inch pieces (1 cup)

1 crimson bell pepper, seeds removed and thinly sliced

1 small chili or jalapeño pepper, seeds eliminated and thinly sliced

14 oz. Lite coconut milk (1 can)

2 cups bird broth

Juice of 1 lime

Handful cilantro leaves (non-compulsory)

Directions:

1. Season the sliced chook breast generously with salt and pepper.

2. In a gigantic (5-6 quart) soup pot, warmth the coconut oil over excessive heat and add the hen breast. Stir-fry over excessive warmth for 4-5 minutes, or until the hen is not pink on the external.

3. Add the sliced onion, minced garlic, and minced ginger and proceed to stir-fry for an additional 2-3 minutes.

4. Include the cubed pumpkin and diced zucchini, and mix. Add the sliced bell pepper, sliced chili or jalapeño pepper, coconut milk, fowl broth, and lime juice.

5. Stir the whole thing together.

6. Deliver to a boil, then lessen the heat, cover, and enable to simmer for approximately 20 minutes, or until the pumpkin is entirely cooked.

7. Use additional salt and pepper to season, if desired. Garnish with cilantro leaves to serve.

Mustard Baked Chicken Tenders

This mustard baked hen tenders recipe is outstanding simple and deliciously spicy. The mustard sauce is ideal over rice or a salad.

Serving: 6

Preparation Time: 5 Minutes

Cook Time: 30 Minutes

Total Time: 35 Minutes

Ingredients:

1 lbs. Hen tenders

½ cup whole grain mustard

2 tbsp. Chopped recent tarragon

½ oz. Lemon juice

1 clove garlic, minced

½ tsp. Paprika, candy smoked if you have it

½ tsp. Pepper

¼ tsp. Kosher salt

additional tarragon to garnish (optional)

Directions:

1. Preheat oven to 425F (220C)

2. Combine all parts, besides hen tenders, in a massive bowl and blend good.

3. Add bird and blend to coat with the mustard sauce.

4. Place chook and sauce into a large baking dish and cover.

5. Bake except fowl has cooked by means of, 15 to 20 minutes.

6. To assess the doneness of the chicken tenders, cut one halfway by means of.

7. If the juices are clear and the meat appears carried out, it's equipped.

Prosciutto Wrapped Chicken Breast with Cream Cheese

Fowl breast wrapped in cream cheese and prosciutto is an amazingly clean and healthful way to bake an appropriate juicy and delicious bird breast.

Serving: 3

Preparation Time: 10 Minutes

Cook Time: 30 Minutes

Total Time: 40 Minutes

Ingredients:

1 chicken breast

1.Four oz. Finely sliced prosciutto (Parma ham)

1.3 oz. Cream cheese (low-fats)

5-10 contemporary basil leaves (depending on measurement)

Pepper

Directions:

1. Situation the prosciutto slices on a piece of aluminum foil so the sides overlap fairly.

2. Unfold the cream cheese evenly onto the prosciutto. Professional TIP: Take the cream cheese out of the fridge quarter-hour earlier than you start utilizing it to let it heat up a bit.

3. A good way to make it a lot less difficult to work with.

4. Location the contemporary basil leaves on prime in order that they quilt the cream cheese.

5. Gently, wrap the prosciutto, cream cheese, and basil leaves around the fowl breast and grind just a little pepper on prime (or a variety of pepper if you're like me and love pepper).

6. Bake the Prosciutto Wrapped chook Breast with Cream Cheese within the oven for 25-30 minutes (depending on how massive the chicken breast is) at 380 F (one hundred ninety C).

7. Let the chook leisure for a minute outside the over earlier than reducing and serving. Revel in!

Instant Pot Chicken Chili

This on the spot pot hen chili is an easy green chili (chile verde) without beans effortlessly made inside the instantaneous pot!

Serving: 6

Preparation Time: 10 Minutes

Cook Time: 30 Minutes

Total Time: 40 Minutes

Ingredients:

1 tbsp. Vegetable oil

1 yellow onion, diced

four cloves garlic, minced

1 tsp. Floor cumin

1 tsp. Oregano

2½ lbs. Bird breasts, boneless & skinless

sixteen oz. Salsa verde

Toppings

2 applications queso fresco , crumbled (or sour cream)

2 avocados, diced

eight radishes, chopped high-quality

8 springs cilantro (optional)

Directions:

1. Set the immediate Pot to the sauté atmosphere, medium.

2. Add the vegetable oil.

3. Add the onion and cook for three minutes, stirring most commonly until the onion starts to soften.

4. Add the garlic, and stir for one more minute.

5. Add the cumin and oregano and stir for an additional minute.

6. Pour ½ of the salsa verde into the pot. High with the chook breasts and pour the rest salsa verde over the chook.

7. Location the lid on the instantaneous Pot and set to "manual". Rotate the stopwatch for 10 minutes.

8. Use a common free up (let the on the spot Pot liberate the pressure through itself).

9. As soon as whole, eliminate the chicken from the pot and shred the chook with a fork.

10. Return the fowl to the pot and stir to combine.

11. Serve in a bowl with the toppings or use for tacos.

12. Further instantaneous Pot bird Chili can be frozen in an airtight container.

Healthy Homemade Chicken Nuggets

These healthful homemade chook Nuggets taste so excellent you won't feel they're definitely good for you! They're low-carb, grain-free, and include handiest six parts.

Serving: 4

Preparation Time: 10 Minutes

Cook Time: 40 Minutes

Total Time: 50 Minutes

Ingredients:

2 hen breasts, boneless and skinless

½ cup almond flour

1 tbsp. Italian seasoning

2 tbsp. Put some virgin olive oil

½ tsp. Salt

½ tsp. Pepper

Directions:

1. Preheat oven to four hundred F (200 C). Put together a huge baking sheet with parchment paper.

2. In a bowl, stir collectively the almond flour, Italian seasoning, salt, and pepper.

3. Cut any final fats off the fowl breasts and discard. Then slice into 1-inch thick portions.

4. Spray the chicken slices with some virgin olive oil.

5. Place every piece into the bowl with the flour and canopy liberally. Then place on the baking sheet.

6. Bake for 20 minutes, then flip the broiler on and location under the broiler three-4 minutes to make the outside crispy.

7. Serve immediately with mustard or scorching sauce.

Crockpot Ranch Chicken

This crockpot ranch fowl is straightforward, soul-satisfying, and just the type of healthful low-carb consolation food you want after a long day!

Serving: 6

Preparation Time: 10 Minutes

Cook Time: 4 Hours, 20 Minutes

Total Time: 4 Hours, 30 Minutes

Ingredients:

4 chicken breasts boneless, skinless

½ cup low sodium chook inventory

1 cup chive and onion cream cheese spread

1 1-oz. Bundle ranch dressing and seasoning mix

½ tsp. Black pepper freshly floor

Directions:

1. To brown the fowl (non-compulsory): in case your crockpot has a saute atmosphere, spray the inside with cooking spray and set to saute.

2. If your crockpot does not have a saute surroundings, spray a skillet with cooking spray and heat over medium-excessive heat.

3. Blot the chicken dry with a paper towel and add to the crockpot or skillet. Cook for three - 5 minutes or until the hen is calmly browned. Flip and repeat on the opposite facet.

4. If utilizing a skillet to brown the chook, transfer the fowl breasts to the crockpot after browning.

5. Include the fowl stock, pepper, cream cheese, and ranch dressing mix. Quilt and prepare dinner on low warmness for four hours or until the fowl is cooked through and reaches an inside temperature of 165 F (seventy four C).

6. When the bird is cooked, get rid of the chook from the crockpot and whisk the sauce except it is soft. For a thicker sauce, return the crockpot to the saute atmosphere (excessive if possible) and prepare dinner, whisking most often for 5 to 10 minutes.

7. If your crockpot does not have a saute setting, pour the sauce right into a saucepan and warmness over medium-excessive warmth, whisking mostly until the sauce thickens to the favored consistency.

8. Garnish with the publisher 1st baron verulam and sliced inexperienced onions before serving if preferred.

Chicken Cauliflower Casserole (Low Carb)

Chook cauliflower casserole is an easy-to-make dish that is high in protein whilst being low in carbs, energy, and fat. it makes for the correct healthful dinner preference!

Serving: 5

Preparation Time: 10 Minutes

Cook Time: 40 Minutes

Total Time: 50 Minutes

Ingredients:

1 lb. Cooked bird, shredded

1 red bell pepper, diced

1 inexperienced bell pepper, diced

2 cups salsa

three cups cauliflower rice

1 large egg

1/3 cups low-moisture cheddar, shredded

2 tbsp. Low-moisture cheddar, shredded

1 tsp. Cumin

½ tsp. Paprika

Limes & cilantro for topping

Directions:

1. Situation cauliflower rice in a skillet with ¼ cup water. Convey to a medium heat and warmness until softened (about 5 minutes).

2. Preheat oven to 375F (190C) and grease a 7.5x11" baking dish evenly with further virgin olive oil.

3. Get rid of the cauliflower rice from the warmth and drain any excess liquid.

4. Situation the cauliflower in a mixing bowl with the egg and 1/3 cup shredded cheddar. Combine unless the egg and cheese are blended well together.

5. Transfer the cauliflower blend to the all set baking dish and delicate into a good layer.

6. Bake 20-25 minutes at except set (experiment the crust with a type to scan consistency).

Even as the cauliflower bakes, add the bell peppers to a skillet and sauté for four-5 minutes unless tender.

7. Add the shredded chook, paprika, cumin, sautéed bell peppers, and salsa to a mixing bowl and gently combine it all collectively.

8. Once the cauliflower is completed baking, spread the bird blend over the crust and sprinkle the remaining 2 tablespoons of cheese excessive.

9. Bake at 375F for 7 minutes to heat the hen blend and melt the cheese.

10. Serve instantly with limes and cilantro.

Healthy Chicken and Mushroom Skillet

This one-pan wholesome chook and mushroom skillet with kale is ready in just 35 mins with minimal cleanup. The lemony garlicky taste of this dish will have you achieving for seconds!

Serving: 5

Preparation Time: 5 Minutes

Cook Time: 35 Minutes

Total Time: 40 Minutes

Ingredients:

1½ lb. Chicken breast (three or four bird breasts)

2 tsp. Italian seasoning

2 tbsp. Vegetable oil

2 cloves garlic, minced

8 oz. Little one bella (crimini) mushrooms, sliced

6 cups chopped kale leaves, tightly packed (about ½ - ¾ lb kale)

½ cup bird broth or water

Zest and juice of 1 lemon

Salt & pepper to taste

Directions:

1. Season the chicken breasts with Italian seasoning, salt, and pepper.

2. Warmness the vegetable oil in a enormous skillet, and cook the bird breasts over excessive warmth about 5-eight minutes on each part, or until nicely browned.

3. Add the minced garlic and sliced mushrooms to the pan and stir.

4. Add the kale leaves and hen broth. You might have got to add 1/2 the kale leaves, wait except they prepare dinner down, then add the leisure.

5. Flip the warmness down and continue to cook, stirring probably, for about 10 minutes or except the liquid is usually evaporated, the kale is wilted, and the fowl breasts are thoroughly cooked.

6. Optional: situation a couple of lemon halves dealing with down into the skillet in the course of the last couple of minutes of cooking. When they cool, which you can squeeze additional lemon juice over the entire dish for one more zing of flavor

7. Do away with from warmth and stir in the lemon zest and lemon juice. Season with further salt and pepper, if preferred.

Lemon Chicken Piccata

Lemon chook Piccata is a budget-friendly take on an Italian basic! Extremely effortless and low carb, this piccata recipe is one you'll want to make over and over!

Serving: 4

Preparation Time: 10 Minutes

Cook Time: 40 Minutes

Total Time: 50 Minutes

Ingredients:

2 skinless, boneless chicken breasts

three tbsp. Unsalted butter

1½ tbsp. All purpose flour

¼ tsp. White pepper

¼ tsp. Salt

2 tbsp. Olive oil

? Cup dry white wine

? Cup low sodium bird inventory

¼ cup lemon juice

¼ cup drained capers

¼ cup Italian Parsley minced

Salt & pepper

Directions:

1. Slice each and every fowl breasts in half of lengthwise so you get 2 thin bird slices from each and every breast (you can see how they're supposed to look within the second picture on this publish).

2. If the bird slices are very thick, use a mallet or a different heavy object to flatten them relatively - you need them no more than ½ inch (1.25 cm) thick.

3. Spread the flour out thinly on a dinner plate. Add salt and pepper to seasoned. Evenly dredge the hen breast slices within the professional flour, shaking off extra flour. Set apart.

4. Warmness a gigantic saute pan over medium-high warmness. When the oil is shimmering, add the bird breast slices to the pan. Prepare dinner for three -4 minutes until browned.

5. Flip the chicken slices over and brown on the opposite aspect. Dispose of the bird slices from the pan and put aside.

6. Add the wine to the saute pan, stirring and scraping up the browned bits on the bottom of the pan.

7. Add the lemon juice and bird stock. Expand the warmth to high and boil until the sauce thickens - about 3 minutes.

8. Curb the warmness to medium and add the butter.

9. Stir in the capers and parsley and add the chook breast slices again to the pan to rewarm.

10. Taste the sauce and alter the seasoning.

Chicken and Egg Salad

This healthful chicken and egg salad is considered one of my pass-to lunch recipes. It tastes first-rate, is so easy to make that you could slightly call it cooking, and you can make a huge batch and save it within the fridge for days.

Serving: 5

Preparation Time: 10 Minutes

Cook Time: 20 Minutes

Total Time: 30 Minutes

Ingredients:

2 cooked bird breasts

3 rough-boiled eggs

2 tbsp. Fats-free mayo

1 tbsp. Curry powder

Chives or basil (non-compulsory)

Salt (non-compulsory)

Directions:

1. Bake the fowl within the oven at 365 F (185 C) for approximately 20 min (verify with a knife that the bird is cooked all of the method by means of).

2. For good 8 minutes boil the eggs.

3. Reduce fowl and eggs into bite-sized portions.

4. Combine the mayo with curry powder (i like to make use of plenty of curry powder. With 1/2 a tablespoon and taste earlier than including extra).

5. Combine the whole lot in a huge bowl and mix.

6. Let it cool within the fridge for at least 10 minutes (it will get even better if you happen to leave it in the fridge overnight).

7. Serve on toast or truffles with chives and a bit salt on top.

Smothered Creamy Skillet Chicken

This low-carb, high-protein Creamy Skillet Chicken is the perfect mix of healthy and delicious! It's creamy and flavorful while still being healthy and super easy to make.

Serving: 6

Preparation Time: 10 Minutes

Cook Time: 30 Minutes

Total Time: 40 Minutes

Ingredients:

1 lbs. Hen breast

eight oz. Mushrooms, chopped

four cups fresh spinach

four cloves massive garlic, minced

6 inexperienced onions (sometimes called scallions), chopped

7-eight mini candy bell peppers, sliced

2 tsp. Parsley, chopped

1 cup hen or vegetable broth

1 cup unsweetened cashew milk

2 tbsp. Greek yogurt

1 tbsp. cream cheese

2 tsp. Extra virgin olive oil

Salt & pepper to taste

Directions:

1. Add 1 tsp. Olive oil to a tremendous skillet over medium heat.

2. Season hen breasts with salt and pepper. Add to skillet and sauté for three minutes on each and every aspect or until golden brown and practically cooked by means of. Place it aside where safe.

3. In the equal scorching skillet, add closing tsp. Olive oil and shrink warmness.

4. Add garlic and permit to prepare dinner for about 30 seconds.

5. Add inexperienced onion and half of of the broth and raise warmth to medium.

6. Add mushrooms & peppers and deliver to a medium simmer. Cook dinner for five minutes

7. In a separate bowl, whisk yogurt, cashew milk, and 1 tsp. Parsley, then pour into skillet.

8. Add spinach and stir unless mixed.

9. Enable sauce to bubble frivolously with greens, lowering heat if wanted and stirring sometimes, for 5 extra minutes.

10. Nestle fowl breasts into the skillet. Add ultimate broth and mascarpone or cream cheese, and cook for 5-10 minutes unless bird is cooked through and the sauce has thickened.

11. High with closing parsley and serve.

10 Low-Carb Smoothies for Diabetics

Strawberry Banana Protein Smoothie

This cool and fresh Strawberry Banana Protein Smoothie packs 25 grams of protein and is the best method to quiet down with a healthy and scrumptious protein shake after a workout or day in the solar!

Serving: 4

Preparation Time: 5 Minutes

Cook Time: 5 Minutes

Total Time: 10 Minutes

Ingredients:

Four oz. Strawberries

1 oz. Banana

1 scoop vanilla protein powder (1 oz.)

1 tsp. Flaxseed

Water

Directions:

1. Put all the elements in a blender and mixture until utterly mixed (i take advantage of my Nutribullet).

2. Start out with just a little water and then slowly add as a lot as you like to get the correct consistency.

3. Serve over ice or use frozen berries to offer the smoothie a thicker (nearly slush-ice) consistency.

Blueberry Smoothie (Low-Carb, High-Protein)

What would be higher after a workout than this scrumptious low-carb, high protein blueberry smoothie? It could be wealthy and creamy however additionally full of antioxidants!

Serving: 3

Preparation Time: 5 Minutes

Cook Time: 5 Minutes

Total Time: 10 Minutes

Ingredients:

14 oz. Canned unsweetened coconut milk

half cup unsweetened almond milk

half of cup blueberries recent or frozen

4 tbsp. Pea protein powder

half of tsp. Vanilla extract

Directions:

1. Add the entire constituents to a excessive-pace blender and combination on high until tender (should turn a light purple colour).

2. Use a silicon spatula to wipe down the edges if the protein powder gets stuck.

3. Non-compulsory: you can add a bit Stevia or a further no-calorie sweetener if you need your smoothie sweeter.

4. Serve immediately with a straw and experience!

Low-Carb Smoothie Bowl with Berries

This low-carb smoothie bowl with berries is tremendous for a healthful start to your morning. It is a delicious, creamy breakfast it's ready in best 5 minutes.

Serving: 4

Preparation Time: 5 Minutes

Cook Time: 5 Minutes

Total Time: 10 Minutes

Ingredients:

1/2 cup unsweetened almond milk

2 oz. chopped strawberries

3 cups crushed ice

1/3 cup pea protein powder (or vanilla protein powder)

1/2 tsp. psyllium husk powder

1 tbsp. coconut oil

5 - 10 drops liquid Stevia

Directions:

1. Put the ice cubes into your blender and depart them to take a seat for five mins before mixing.

2. This could let them soften barely so that the blender has a few traction to combo them into crushed ice.

3. Upload the rest of the components to the blender and mix till clean, creamy, and light red.

4. Spoon at once into a bowl.

5. Non-compulsory: Garnish with fresh strawberries, coconut flakes, and cocoa nibs to serve.

Raspberry Chocolate Avocado Smoothie

Want a first rate low carb smoothie that doesn't skimp on flavour? This dairy-free Chocolate Avocado Smoothie recipe makes a scrumptious filling snack or healing drink.

Serving: 3

Preparation Time: 5 Minutes

Cook Time: 0 Minutes

Total Time: 5 Minutes

Ingredients:

1 1/4 cup Silk Cashew Milk

half of avocado

1/3 cup frozen raspberries

1 tbsp cocoa powder

Swerve Sweetener to taste (I used 1 tbsp powdered Swerve Sweetener)

1/eight tsp raspberry extract

Directions:

1. You definitely know the preparation. Put all elements in a blender and mixture except tender.

2. For a thinner smoothie, add further 1/four cup cashew milk.

Healthy Strawberry Basil Smoothie

I'm all about the smoothies. This keto Strawberry and Basil Smoothie is delicious for breakfast and if like me you decide on to haven't any sweeteners as good as no sugar, you might like this recipe.Sweetened naturally just with strawberries. It's creamy, it's dreamy and it's additionally dairy free. Consider free so as to add any of the not obligatory extras: MCT oil for additonal fat and energy raise, and collagen or protein powder for added protein to maintain hunger at bay and your blood sugar phases healthy.

Serving: 2

Preparation Time: 5 Minutes

Cook Time: 0 Minutes

Total Time: 5 Minutes

Ingredients:

1 cup chilled strawberries (152 g/ five.4 oz.)

3/four cup 10% fats Greek yogurt or coconut yogurt, e.g. Coyo (188 g/ 6.6 oz.)

10 clean basil leaves

1/2 cup unsweetened almond milk or cashew milk (a hundred and twenty ml/ 4 fl oz.)

2-4 ice cubes commands

Directions:

1. Blitz all the substances together in a excessive pace blender till easy.

2. Add any of the elective extras.

3. Sprinkle with a hint of acai powder for a further antioxidant enhances.

4. Best when served sparkling, however can be stored in the refrigerator for 1 day.

Key Lime Pie Protein Shake

What could be higher than having fun with a bit of key lime pie in a wealthy creamy shake packed with protein!?! This shake makes an pleasant breakfast or snack, and is so delicious that you'll have a hard time believing that it's actually good for you!

Serving: 5

Preparation Time: 5 Minutes

Cook Time: 0 Minutes

Total Time: 5 Minutes

Ingredients:

1/2 cup

fat free cottage cheese [1]

1Scoop vanilla protein powder [2]

1 tbs Lime juice (recent or bottled, I in my view like key lime juice nice!)

5-10 Ice cubes (relying on how thick you adore it, use much less for a thinner consistency)

1/2-1 cupWater (Alter this in keeping with favored consistency)

2-4 pkts Stevia (or 1/four-1 tsp sweetener of option)

2-three drops green food coloring, or a handful of spinach to make it inexperienced!

Not obligatory:

1 tbs sugar free vanilla instantaneous pudding mix

non-compulsory:

half of tsp xanthan gum [3], 1 graham cracker, overwhelmed into crumbs

Directions:

1. The estimated whole time to make this recipe is 5 minutes.

2. Put the whole lot into a blender and combination except creamy consistency is reached!

3. Prime with a beaten graham cracker if preferred!

Cinnamon Roll Smoothie

Wholesome, scrumptious and tastes much like a cinnamon roll.

Serving: 2

Preparation Time: 5 Minutes

Cook Time: 0 Minutes

Total Time: 5 Minutes

Ingredients:

1 cup almond milk

2 tablespoons vanilla protein powder

1/2 teaspoon cinnamon

1/4 teaspoon vanilla extract

4 teaspoons Swervesweetener

1 teaspoon flaxmeal

1 cup ice

Directions:

Pour all ingredients in blender, upload ice final. combination on high for 30 seconds or till completely combined and thickened.

Keto Smoothie - Blueberry

This keto smoothie is superb for a speedy breakfast or a publish-exercise refuel alternative. It's packed with antioxidants for higher cleansing, nutrition c for a healthy immune system, and folate for proper cholesterol operate.

Serving: 3

Preparation Time: 6 Minutes

Cook Time: 0 Minutes

Total Time: 6 Minutes

Ingredients:

1 cup Coconut Milk or almond milk

1/four cup Blueberries

1 tsp Vanilla Extract

1 tsp MCT Oil or coconut oil

30 g Protein Powder non-compulsory

Directions:

Put all of the substances right into a blender, and blend until smooth.

Low Carb Strawberry Cheesecake Smoothie

This low carb strawberry cheesecake smoothie whips up in simply minutes. It's much more delicious than combining your favourite milkshake and cheesecake. I do know from expertise that once dwelling a healthy low carb way of life you could more often than not suppose like your depriving yourself of things you love, like fruity smoothies and wealthy cheesecake. That's why I've created this deliciously healthful smoothie.

Serving: 4

Preparation Time: 5 Minutes

Cook Time: 0 Minutes

Total Time: 5 Minutes

Ingredients:

half cup low-fat cottage cheese

2 oz of cream cheese

half cup strawberries

four tablespoons Swervesweetener

1 cup of ice cubes 2 handfuls

1/4 cup Silk Unsweetened Soy Milk

half of teaspoon natural vanilla extract

Directions:

1. Add all of the components into a blender and blend except tender and conveniently pourable.

2. Style and regulate consistency and sweetness with the aid of including more ice and/or sweetener.

Minty Green Protein Smoothie Shake

Serving: 2

Preparation Time: 10 Minutes

Cook Time: 0 Minutes

Total Time: 10 Minutes

Ingredients:

1/2 avocado

1 cup contemporary spinach

10-12 drops SweetLeaf® Liquid Stevia Peppermint sweet Drops™

1 scoop whey protein powder

half cup unsweetened almond milk

1/four tsp peppermint extract

1 cup ice

Not obligatory: Cacao nibs

Directions:

1. Location avocado, spinach, protein powder and milk in a blender and combination unless smooth.

2. Add the SweetLeaf® Liquid Stevia Peppermint candy Drops™, extract, and ice, and mixture unless thick.

3. Style and alter stevia, as wanted.

18 Tasty Diabetic-Friendly Recipes

Three-Pepper Pizza

Opposite to popular belief, pizza may be a healthy dish. Including vegetables like bell peppers, which can be the quality source of diet C, boosts your veggie consumption. Moreover, if you pick reduced-fats or fats-free cheese you narrow again on fats and nevertheless get a lift of calcium.

Serving: 4

Preparation Time: 10 Minutes

Cook Time: 0 Minutes

Total Time: 10 Minutes

Ingredients:

1/4 teaspoon Italian seasoning

1/3 cup tomato paste

1/four cup water

1 (12-inch) prebaked refrigerated pizza crust

1 cup (4 ounces) shredded part-skim mozzarella cheese

1 half of cups diced green, crimson, and yellow bell pepper (about three small peppers)

half of onion, chopped

Directions:

1. Preheat oven to 450°.

2. Mix seasoning, tomato paste, and water in a small bowl; stir well. Spray on pizza crust. High evenly with cheese. Sprinkle bell pepper and onion evenly over cheese.

3. Bake at 450° for 10 to 12 minutes or except cheese melts. Cut into 6 wedges, and serve.

4. Tip: Bell peppers are available an assortment of colours: inexperienced, crimson, yellow, orange, brown, and purple. The colour relies on form and ripeness. When peppers are picked earlier than they attain maturity, they are inexperienced. However when left on the vine just a little longer, a pepper ripens and changes color, depending on its type.

Seared Chicken with Avocado

Avocados are a fine superfood to add to any meal. They are wealthy in coronary heart-healthy monounsaturated fats, fiber, and vitamin E. Their taste is mild, however provides a creamy texture to the fowl.

Serving: 5

Preparation Time: 5 Minutes

Cook Time: 5 Minutes

Total Time: 10 Minutes

Ingredients:

1 half of teaspoons blackened seasoning

four (4-ounce) skinless, boneless bird breast halves

1 teaspoon olive oil

1 diced peeled avocado

2 tablespoons chopped sparkling cilantro

1 jalapeño pepper, seeded and finely chopped

2 tablespoons clean lime juice (about 1 lime)

1/four teaspoon salt

1 lime, reduce into fourths

Directions:

1. Sprinkle seasoning on each aspects of fowl. Warm oil in a large nonstick skillet over excessive warmth.

2. Add chook to pan, easy side down; prepare dinner 1 minute or until seared.

3. reduce warmness to medium; cook dinner 3 mins on each side or until gently browned.

4. Integrate avocado, cilantro, pepper, lime juice, and salt. Squeeze one-fourth lime over every piece of fowl earlier than serving.

5. Serve with avocado aggregate.

Cumin Quick Bread

Serve this cumin bread with dinner or for breakfast, with Smart Balance butter unfold for a lift of omega-three fatty acids

Serving: 8

Preparation Time: 5 Minutes

Cook Time: 5 Minutes

Total Time: 10 Minutes

Ingredients:

1 1/2 cups all-cause flour

2 tablespoons "measures-like-sugar" calorie-loose sweetener

1 tablespoon baking powder

2 teaspoons floor cumin

half teaspoon cumin seed, barely crushed

1/four teaspoon dry mustard

1/four teaspoon salt

2/3 cup fats-unfastened milk

1/three cup egg replacement

2 half of tablespoons vegetable oil

2 tablespoons picante sauce

Cooking spray

Directions:

1. Preheat oven to 350°.

2. Integrate first 7 substances in a medium bowl; make a properly in middle of combination.

3. Integrate milk and subsequent 3 elements; stir well.

4. Add to flour aggregate, stirring simply till dry ingredients are moistened.

5. Spoon batter into an eight half- x 4 1/2-inch loafpan coated with cooking spray.

6. Bake at 350° for 40 minutes or till a wooden choose inserted in center comes out easy.

7. put off from pan, and allow cool on a wire rack.

Apple Slaw

This guilt-free aspect is sweetened with apples and even has fiber, to help indigestion. Serve at your subsequent picnic rather of fatty potato salad and wow the group.

Serving: 8

Preparation Time: 5 Minutes

Cook Time: 0 Minutes

Total Time: 5 Minutes

Directions:

1. Mix first 7 materials in a tremendous bowl, stirring with a whisk unless blended.

2. Add cabbage and apple; toss well.

3. Cover and kick back completely, tossing on occasion.

4. If you want to add a bit of extra tartness to this salad, you could make it with Granny Smith apples.

Beef Kebabs

This grilled dish is exceptional any time of the yr. it's colorful vegetables are filled with vitamins like diet C, fiber and nutrition E. pork is chock complete of vitamin B12 and iron. do this kebab with chicken for a leaner opportunity.

Serving: 5

Preparation Time: 5 Minutes

Cook Time: 0 Minutes

Total Time: 5 Minutes

Ingredients:

(1-pound) meat tenderloin

2 teaspoons Worcestershire sauce

1 medium-estimate green chime pepper, cut into 20 squares

10 cherry tomatoes

10 little mushrooms

2 little yellow squash, cut into 10 cuts

1/8 teaspoon dark pepper

Cooking splash

1/4 teaspoon salt

Directions:

1. Get ready flame broil.

2. Cut meat into 20 (3/4-inch) 3D squares. Spray Worcestershire sauce on the meat. String meat, chime pepper, tomatoes, mushrooms, and squash on the other hand onto 5 (12-inch) sticks.

3. Sprinkle equally with dark pepper.

4. Spot kebabs on flame broil rack covered with cooking splash; barbecue, revealed, 10 minutes or to wanted level of doneness, turning once. Sprinkle equitably with salt.

5. Tip: If utilizing wooden sticks, make sure to absorb them water 30 minutes before stringing to shield them from consuming amid flame broiling.

Basil Scallops with Spinach Fettuccine

Spinach fettuccine is a tasty method to get in your veggie servings. Tossed with scallops, this dish a pleasant source of nutrition B12 and protein. You would be able to also replace chicken, which is additionally a lean source of protein.

Serving: 6

Preparation Time: 15 Minutes

Cook Time: 0 Minutes

Total Time: 15 Minutes

Ingredients:

Eight ounces raw spinach fettuccine

1 half pounds sea scallops

three/four teaspoon freshly ground black pepper

Cooking spray

2 tablespoons extravirgin olive oil

1 tablespoon Dijon mustard

1 tablespoon chopped fresh basil

1/4 teaspoon salt

3/4 cup dry white wine or low-sodium bird broth

1/three cup finely chopped green onion (about 2)

3 tablespoons chopped contemporary parsley

Directions:

1. Cook dinner pasta in line with bundle instructions, omitting salt and fats. Drain.

2. Rinse scallops, and pat dry with a paper towel. Spray with pepper the scallops. Situation a massive nonstick skillet coated with cooking spray over medium-high warmth except hot.

3. add half of scallops; prepare dinner 3 minutes on each and every part or except finished.

4. Dispose of scallops from pan; preserve warm. Repeat approach with final scallops.

5. Combine olive oil and next 3 components; put aside.

6. Position same pan over high heat except sizzling. Add wine and inexperienced onions, and prepare dinner 1 minute.

7. Add olive oil combo; cook dinner 15 seconds.

8. Add scallops and any gathered juices; cook 15 seconds, stirring always. Juices over pasta and spoon scallops.

9. Sprinkle with parsley.

Snapper with Tomato-Caper Topping

Halibut, sea bass, redfish, or pompano may also paintings properly on this recipe.

Serving: 6

Preparation Time: 20 Minutes

Cook Time: 0 Minutes

Total Time: 20 Minutes

Ingredients:

2 cups halved grape tomatoes

2 tablespoons capers, drained

 2 tablespoons contemporary lemon juice (about 1 lemon)

2 teaspoons olive oil

1 half of teaspoons dried or 1 tablespoon chopped recent basil

1/4 teaspoon salt

1/eight teaspoon beaten purple pepper (not obligatory)

four (6-ounce) snapper or grouper fillets (about 3/four inch thick)

Cooking spray

1 teaspoon paprika

2 tablespoons chopped fresh parsley

1 lemon, reduce into four wedges

Directions:

1. Preheat oven to 450º.

2. Mix first 6 ingredients and beaten crimson pepper, if preferred; set aside.

3. Place snapper on a broiler pan lined with aluminum foil; coat foil with cooking spray.

 4. Sprinkle snapper with paprika; coat with cooking spray.

5. Bake at 450º for 10 minutes.

6. Prime snapper with tomato combination; bake 5 minutes or until fish flakes readily when verified with a fork.

7. Spray with parsley before serving with lemon wedges.

Deep-Dish Taco Pizza

This household-interesting dish is a go between a pizza and a casserole, and guaranteed to please even the pickiest of eaters. Combine Italian and Mexican cuisines with this dish. Prime with shredded lettuce and diced tomatoes to add some veggies to your pizza.

Serving: 6

Preparation Time: 10 Minutes

Cook Time: 20 Minutes

Total Time: 30 Minutes

Ingredients:

1 pound ground spherical

1/2 cup frozen chopped onion

1 (15-ounce) can diced tomatoes with inexperienced chiles, drained

1 teaspoon salt-free Mexican seasoning

1 (10-ounce) can refrigerated pizza crust dough

Cooking spray

1 cup (4 oz.) shredded decreased-fat sharp Cheddar or part-skim mozzarella cheese

Salsa (non-compulsory)

decreased-fat sour cream (optionally available)

Directions:

1. Preheat oven to 425°.

2. Cook dinner red meat and onion in a big nonstick skillet over medium-excessive warmth till pork is browned, stirring to collapse. Drain nicely, and return beef combination to pan. Stir in tomatoes and seasoning; cook over medium-excessive warmth 1 minute or until very well heated; set apart.

3. Uncover pizza crust dough. Press into bottom and midway up aspects of a 13 x 9-inch baking dish covered with cooking spray. Spoon pork aggregate over pizza crust dough.

4. Bake at 425° for 12 mins. pinnacle with cheese, and bake 5 minutes or till cheese melts and edges of crust are browned. Remain standing for about 5 minutes before cutting. Serve when it is still hot. top with salsa and sour cream, if favored.

Potato Cakes

These versatile mashed potato patties complement an array of toppings from veggies to veal. And so they're a designated substitute to noodles, rice, and bread.

Serving: 2

Preparation Time: 10 Minutes

Cook Time: 10 Minutes

Total Time: 20 Minutes

Ingredients:

2 (1-pound, 4-ounce) packages refrigerated mashed potatoes (including actually Potatoes)

1 tablespoon dried minced onion

half of teaspoon pepper

1 cup matzo meal

Cooking spray

Directions:

1. Integrate first four components in a large bowl.

2. Divide combination into sixteen quantities, the usage of approximately 1/three cup in each element. Pat each component right into a four-inch diameter cake; place on wax paper.

3. Warmness a massive nonstick skillet over medium-excessive warmness.

4. Coat each aspects of each cake with cooking spray; region in batches in pan. Reduce warmth to medium; prepare dinner 1 to two minutes on each facet or till browned.

5. Put off from pan, and location on wax paper.

Chili-Fried Potatoes

Serve these spicy potatoes with eggs as a homefries dish or in an omelet. Cut out the cheese to get rid of saturated fat.

Serving: 5

Preparation Time: 10 Minutes

Cook Time: 10 Minutes

Total Time: 20 Minutes

Ingredients:

three cups cubed unpeeled baking potato (approximately 1 pound)

1/2 teaspoon olive oil Olive oil-flavored

cooking spray

1 small onion, halved, thinly sliced, and separated into rings

1 teaspoon chili powder

1/four teaspoon salt

half of cup (2 ounces) shredded decreased-fat sharp Cheddar cheese

Directions:

1. Set up potato in a steamer basket over boiling water. cover and steam 10 mins or till tender. remove from warmness.

2. Warmth oil in a big nonstick skillet lined with cooking spray over medium-excessive warmness.

3. Add onion; sauté 3 minutes or until soft. upload potato, chili powder, and salt.

4. Cook dinner five minutes or till potato is lightly browned, stirring frequently.

5. The potato can be sprinkle with cheese. Cover, remove from warmth, and permit stand 1 minute or till cheese melts.

Cantaloupe Sherbet

This effortless 5-ingredient melon sherbet is a pleasant method to transform fresh cantaloupe right into a low-sugar frozen dessert.

You more commonly is not going to to find this sherbet flavor at any ice cream parlor. Do that vitamin-C rich canteloupe recipe and experience a guilt-free summer treat.

Serving: 6

Preparation Time: 10 Minutes

Cook Time: 10 Minutes

Total Time: 20 Minutes

Ingredients:

1 big ripe cantaloupe, peeled and finely chopped (about 5 cups)

1/three cup "measures-like-sugar" calorie-loose sweetener

2 tablespoons lemon juice

2 teaspoons unflavored gelatin

1/4 cup bloodless water

1 (8-ounce) carton vanilla fat-unfastened yogurt sweetened with aspartame Cantaloupe wedge (optionally available)

Directions:

1. Integrate cantaloupe, sweetener, and lemon juice in a blender or food processor; process until clean. switch combination to a medium bowl.

2. Sprinkle gelatin over cold water in a small saucepan; allow stand 1 minute. prepare dinner over low heat, stirring till gelatin dissolves, approximately four mins. upload to cantaloupe mixture, stirring properly. add yogurt, stirring till easy.

3. Pour mixture into an eight-inch rectangular pan; freeze till almost firm.

4. Switch mixture to a large bowl; beat with a mixer at high pace until fluffy. Spoon combination again into pan; freeze till company.

5. Scoop into 5 man or woman serving dishes to serve. Garnish each serving with a cantaloupe wedge, if preferred (cantaloupe wedge no longer blanketed in evaluation).

Cookies 'n' Cream Crunch

This 4-ingredient dessert comes collectively swiftly then units in your freezer overnight. Preserve these constituents on hand for these moments when you realize you want a scrumptious dessert for the morning's work birthday gathering or the next day to come's regional block occasion.

Serving: 10

Preparation Time: 20 Minutes

Cook Time: 0 Minutes

Total Time: 20 Minutes

Ingredients:

1 (6 half of-ounce) bundle sugar-free chocolate sandwich cookies, overwhelmed

1/three cup chopped pecans

3 tablespoons decreased-calorie margarine, melted

1 quart vanilla no-sugar-delivered, fats-unfastened ice cream, softened

Directions:

1. Combine first 3 elements; reserve 1 cup mixture. Press closing crumb aggregate firmly in backside of a 9-inch square pan. Freeze 10 minutess.

2. Unfold ice cream over crumb mixture in pan. Sprinkle reserved crumb aggregate over ice cream; gently press

combination into ice cream. Cover and freeze at the least eight hours.

3. To serve, allow stand at room temperature 5 minutes; cut into nine squares.

Fresh Berries with Maple Cream

Recent berries get a refreshing topper. Simply by way of stirring a bit of maple syrup into bitter cream, you get a sweet, creamy sauce that's uncommon over any type of recent fruit.

Don't stress about pleasing your guests with this dessert. It's handy, fast, and low-calorie. Fruits, particularly berries, are a first-class source of sickness-combating antioxidants.

Serving: 8

Preparation Time: 10 Minutes

Cook Time: 0 Minutes

Total Time: 10 Minutes

Ingredients:

3/4 cup fats-free bitter cream

1/4 cup maple syrup 1 cup fresh blueberries

1 half cups fresh raspberries

Directions:

1. Combine butter cream and maple syrup in a small bowl; stir with a whisk.

2. Join berries, and spoon into treat dishes; pour maple cream over berries.

Simple Veggie Tostadas

The quandary along with your weekly Mexican tostada night is that the dish is as a rule high in fats, energy, and sodium. However it doesn't need to be. Here's a high-quality healthy recipe that accommodates the scrumptious Mexican flavors you like whilst cutting the grease and the caloric punch.

Serving: 5

Preparation Time: 10 Minutes

Cook Time: 20 Minutes

Total Time: 30 Minutes

Ingredients:

Cooking spray

2 cups sliced mushrooms

2 small zucchini, sliced

1 colossal red bell pepper, chopped 4

Directions:

1. Position a medium nonstick skillet lined with cooking spray over medium-excessive warmth unless sizzling.

2. Add bell pepper to pan, mushrooms, zucchini.

3. Sauté 3 to five minutes or until veggies are smooth.

4. Spoon about 3/4 cup vegetable combo over black bean blend on each and every tostada.

5. Prime with lettuce, salsa, and cheese.

Barley and Black Bean Salad

Beans and barley are great sources of dietary fiber. Fiber aids in digestion and maintains you feeling full so you may not snack throughout the day.

Serving: 6

Preparation Time: 5 Minutes

Cook Time: 15 Minutes

Total Time: 20 Minutes

Ingredients:

1 field uncooked speedy cooking pearl grain

1 (15-ounce) can darkish beans, washed and depleted

1 pint grape or cherry tomatoes, halved

half of cup finely chopped green bell pepper

half of cup (2 oz) Monterey Jack cheese with jalapeño peppers, cut into 1/4-inch cubes

1/three cup lemon juice

2 tablespoons olive oil

1 teaspoon salt

3/four cup recent cilantro leaves (non-compulsory)

1/8 teaspoon ground red pepper (now not compulsory)

Directions:

1. Prepare dinner barley in keeping with package deal instructional substances, omitting salt.

2. Drain barley in a colander, and rinse with bloodless water unless thoroughly cooled.

3. Mix black beans, subsequent 6 elements, and, if preferred, cilantro and red pepper in a medium bowl.

4. Upload grain to dark bean combo; hurl tenderly.

Honey Grapefruit with Banana

No have to cut out sweets whilst observing your weight! Fruit is a high-quality substitute to more fattening candy treats, and it presents diet C and fiber. Bananas are an excellent source of potassium, to boot.

Serving: 5

Preparation Time: 10 Minutes

Cook Time: 0 Minutes

Total Time: 10 Minutes

Ingredients:

1 (24-ounce) jar refrigerated crimson grapefruit sections (about 2 cups)

1 cup sliced banana (about 1)

1 tablespoon contemporary chopped mint

 1 tablespoon honey

Directions:

1. Channel grapefruit segments, holding 1/4 container juice.

2. Combine grapefruit sections, juice, and last elements in a medium bowl.

3. 2. Hurl delicately to coat. Serve instantly, or quilt and kick back.

Applesauce Pancakes

These diabetic-friendly pancakes are low in fat and easy to make. Serve with clean fruit to make it extra filling, or add fruit proper into the batter. For a coronary heart-healthful complete wheat choice, use complete wheat flour.

Serving: 8

Preparation Time: 15 Minutes

Cook Time: 0 Minutes

Total Time: 15 Minutes

Ingredients:

1 cup all-motive flour

1 teaspoon baking soda

1/8 teaspoon salt

2 tablespoons toasted wheat germ

1 cup nonfat buttermilk

1/4 cup unsweetened applesauce

2 teaspoons vegetable oil

1 colossal egg, calmly crushed

Cooking spray

Sugar-free maple syrup (optional)

recent fruit slices (non-compulsory)

Directions:

1. Mix first four components in a medium bowl; make a good in core of combination. Mix buttermilk and next 3 elements. Add buttermilk mixture to dry materials, stirring just unless dry parts are moistened.

2. Warmth a nonstick griddle or nonstick skillet covered with cooking spray over medium heat. For each pancake, pour 1/4 cup batter onto scorching griddle, spreading to a 5-inch circle. Cook pancakes until tops are blanketed with bubbles and edges appear cooked; turn pancakes, and cook other facet.

3. Serve with maple syrup and fresh fruit, if desired (syrup and fruit no longer incorporated in evaluation).

4. Tip: One tablespoon of sugar-free maple syrup has 8 energy and 3 grams of carbohydrate.

Veggie Sausage-Cheddar Frittata

Vegetable sausage is simpler to crumble if you happen to microwave it at excessive for 15 seconds. Fritattas are a good way to get a form of vitamins and minerals. Eggs and cheese are a best supply of calcium and protein. Mix in veggies to get an antioxidant kick as good as fiber. Fat-free cheese is a healthful substitute, particularly since there's fats within the eggs and sausage.

Serving: 5

Preparation Time: 20 Minutes

Cook Time: 0 Minutes

Total Time: 20 Minutes

Ingredients:

Cooking spray

1 green bell pepper, chopped

1 (eight-ounce) bundle presliced mushrooms

4 (1.3-ounce) frozen vegetable protein sausage patties, thawed and crumbled

1/8 teaspoon salt

1/eight teaspoon freshly floor black pepper

1 cup egg alternative

1/4 cup fats-loose 1/2-and-1/2

1/2 cup (2 oz) shredded reduced-fats sharp Cheddar cheese

Directions:

1. Preheat broiler.

2. Place a 12-inch ovenproof nonstick skillet over medium-high warmness. Coat dish with cooking splash. add chopped bell pepper and mushrooms; sauté 3 mins. add sausage, salt, and pepper; reduce warmness to medium-low, and cook 1 minute.

3. Combine egg replacement and half of-and-1/2; carefully pour over sausage mixture. cover and cook dinner 6 mins. (Frittata could be barely moist on top.) Sprinkle Sprinkle with cheddar.

4. Broil 1 to two minutes or until cheese melts. reduce into eight wedges.

Peanut Butter-and-Jelly Sandwich Cookies

Peanut butter cookies make the ultimate base for a layer of candy strawberry spread. Serve these candy-and-salty cookies for an afternoon snack or a sweet lunchbox surprise.

Serving: 15

Preparation Time: 10 Minutes

Cook Time: 30 Minutes

Total Time: 40 Minutes

Ingredients:

1/4 glass margarine, mellowed

1/4 glass no-sugar-included rich nutty spread

1/2 glass "measures-like-sugar" without calorie sugar

1/4 cup sugar 2 massive egg whites

1 teaspoon vanilla extract

1 three/4 cups all-purpose flour

1 teaspoon baking soda

1/8 teaspoon salt

Cooking spray

three/4 cup low-sugar strawberry spread

Directions:

1. Preheat oven to 350°.

2. Beat margarine and peanut butter with a mixer at medium velocity unless creamy. Step by step add sweetener and sugar, beating well. Include egg whites and vanilla; beat well. Mix flour, soda, and salt in a small bowl, stirring well. Regularly add flour combo to creamed blend, beating well.

3. Form dough into 40 (1-inch) balls. Position balls 2 inches aside on baking sheets lined with cooking spray. Flatten cookies into 2-inch circles utilizing a flat-bottomed glass. Bake at 350° for 8 minutes or until frivolously browned. Cool somewhat on pans; dispose of, and let cool entirely on wire racks.

4. Spread about 1 half of teaspoons strawberry spread on the bottom of each and every of 20 cookies; high with final cookies.

THE END

Author's Notes

Thank you once again for reading!

I would such as you to share your reviews along with your favorite retailer!

Becky Ramos, California, U.S.A

www.ingramcontent.com/pod-product-compliance
Lightning Source LLC
Chambersburg PA
CBHW020316290526
45785CB00007B/2815